THE
ACCUMULAT⏱R
THE REVOLUTIONARY 30-DAY FITNESS PLAN

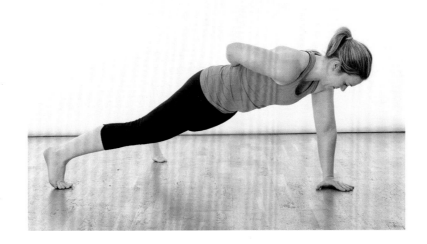

Bloomsbury Sport
An imprint of Bloomsbury Publishing Plc

50 Bedford Square	1385 Broadway
London	New York
WC1B 3DP	NY 10018
UK	USA

www.bloomsbury.com

BLOOMSBURY and the Diana logo are trademarks of
Bloomsbury Publishing Plc

The Accumulator logo is a registered trademark.

First published 2016

© Paul Mumford, 2016

Paul Mumford has asserted his right under the Copyright, Designs and
Patents Act, 1988, to be identified as Author of this work.

All rights reserved. No part of this publication may be reproduced or
transmitted in any form or by any means, electronic or mechanical,
including photocopying, recording, or any information storage or retrieval
system, without prior permission in writing from the publishers.

No responsibility for loss caused to any individual or organization acting on
or refraining from action as a result of the material in this publication can
be accepted by Bloomsbury or the author.

British Library Cataloguing-in-Publication Data
A catalogue record for this book is available from the British Library.

Library of Congress Cataloguing-in-Publication data has been applied for.

ISBN: PB: 978-1-4729-1894-9
      ePDF: 978-1-4729-1896-3
      ePub: 978-1-4729-1895-6

2 4 6 8 10 9 7 5 3 1

Typeset in the UK by Louise Turpin.

ACKNOWLEDGEMENTS
Cover photographs: © EddieMacdonald, 2016
Inside photographs: © EddieMacdonald, 2016, © Shutterstock,
© Getty Images, © Paul Mumford
Art editor: Louise Turpin
Printed and bound in China by C&C Offset Printing Co., Ltd
Bloomsbury Publishing Plc makes every effort to ensure that the papers
used in the manufacture of our books are natural, recyclable products made
from wood grown in well-managed forests. Our manufacturing processes
conform to the environmental regulations of the country of origin.

To find out more about our authors and books visit www.bloomsbury.com.
Here you will find extracts, author interviews, details of forthcoming events
and the option to sign up for our newsletters.

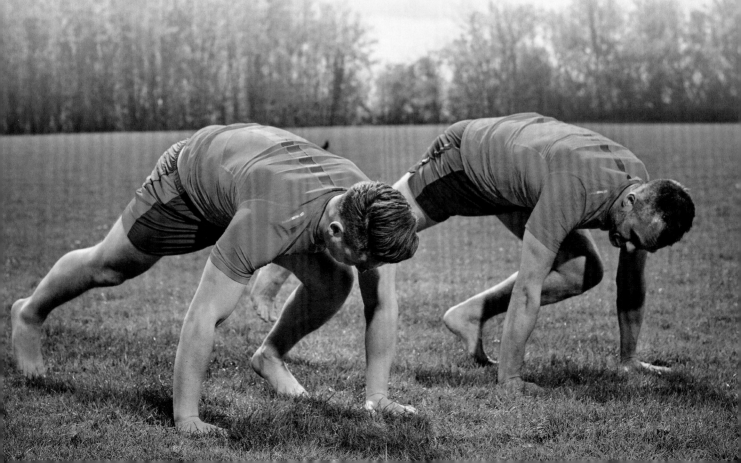

THE
ACCUMULAT⦾R

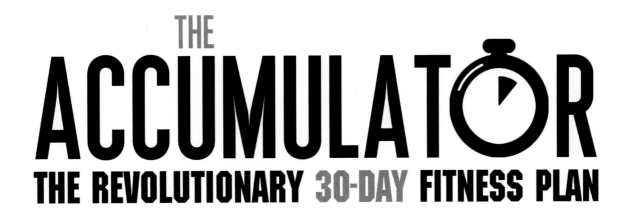

THE REVOLUTIONARY 30-DAY FITNESS PLAN

PAUL MUMFORD

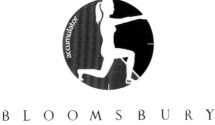

B L O O M S B U R Y
LONDON · NEW DELHI · NEW YORK · SYDNEY

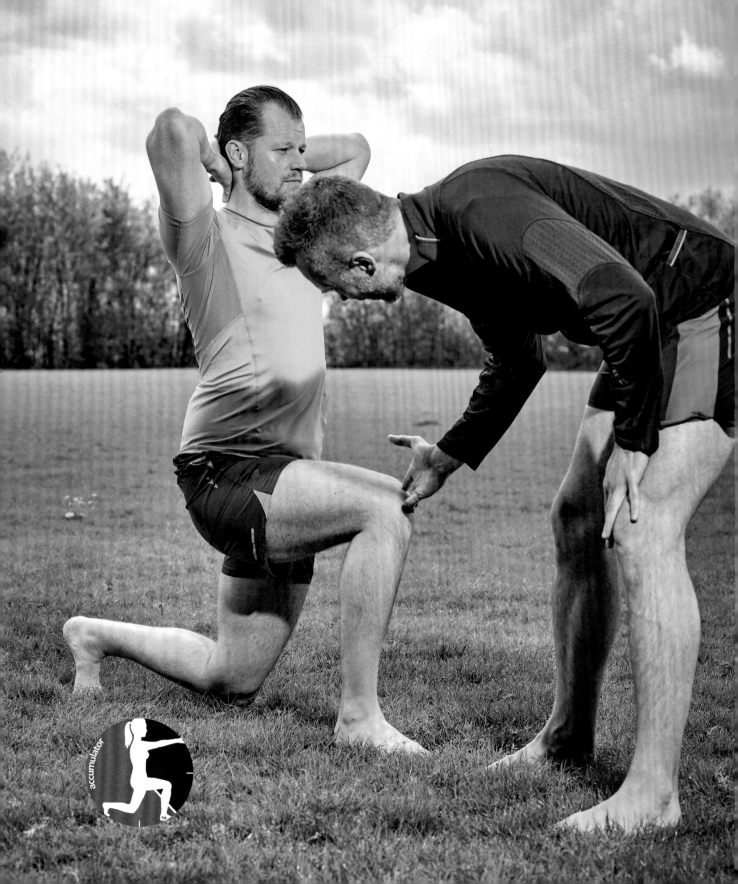

CONTENTS

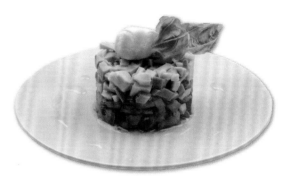

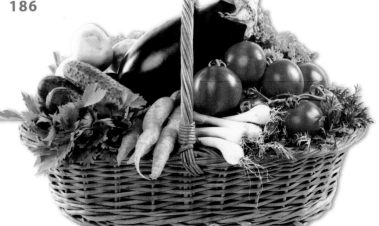

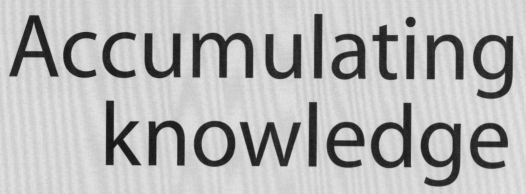

Accumulating knowledge

GREEK PHILOSOPHER PLATO SAID THAT *"HUMAN BEHAVIOUR FLOWS FROM 3 MAIN SOURCES: DESIRE, EMOTION AND KNOWLEDGE".*

YOU ALREADY HAVE THE DESIRE AND EMOTION, SO LET'S START BY DISCOVERING HOW THE ACCUMULATOR™ CAME TO BE AND HOW IT CAN WORK TO CHANGE YOUR LIFE FOR THE BETTER.

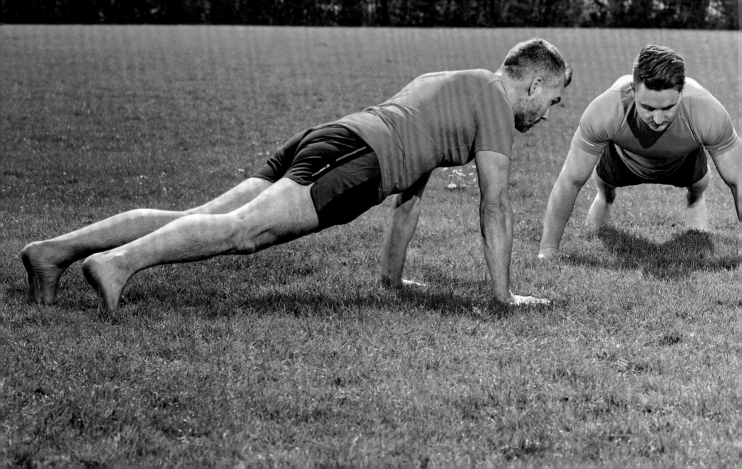

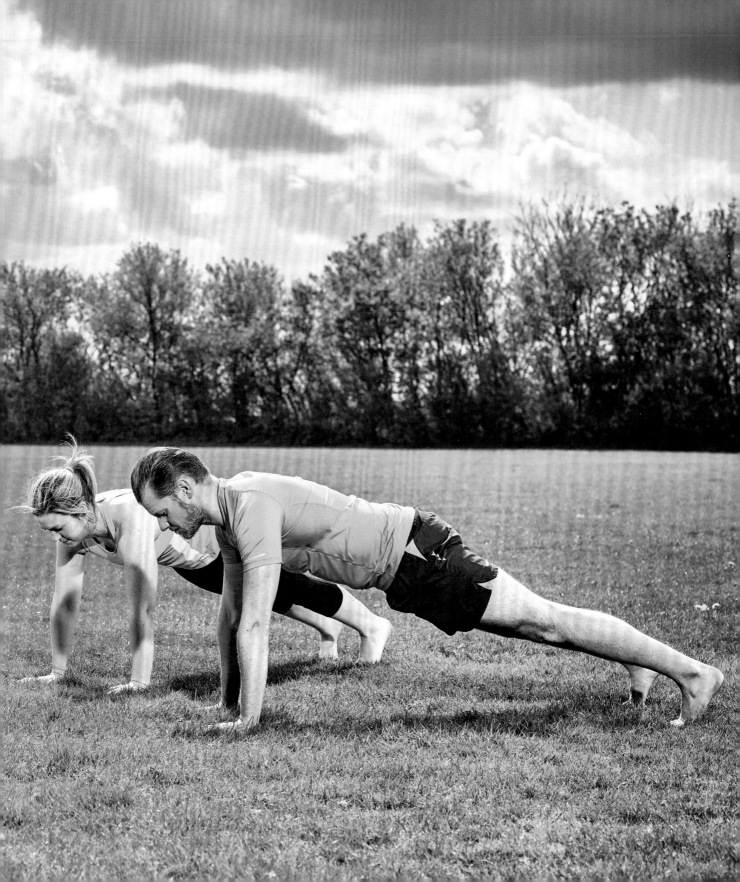

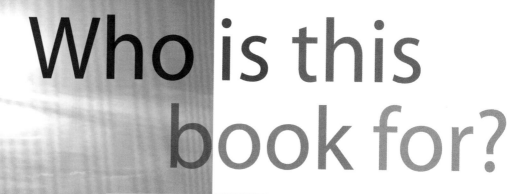

Who is this book for?

AS A SPECIES WE HAVE EVOLVED OVER MILLIONS OF YEARS TO BECOME THE MOST DOMINANT FORCE ON THIS PLANET. OUR BODIES ARE CAPABLE OF MANY INCREDIBLE THINGS – WE HAVE ALL THE EQUIPMENT WITHIN US TO ENABLE US TO RUN LONG DISTANCES, LIFT AND CARRY HEAVY LOADS, CLIMB TO THE HIGHEST POINTS ON EARTH, PUSH, PULL, JUMP, TWIST, SHIFT AND MOVE IN MYRIAD OF AMAZING WAYS. WE HAVE LEARNT TO SURVIVE ON FOOD PROVIDED BY NATURE AND HOW TO THRIVE IN THE MOST INHOSPITABLE ENVIRONMENTS.

Despite all of this, we have become victims of our own success. In the modern world, the human race does not need to do many of the incredible things our bodies are built for because we have invented gadgets to do it for us. We feed ourselves on products created in laboratories and rely less and less on the natural food our bodies are used to and have evolved to thrive upon. As a result, our bodies no longer work as they were intended to and, as a species, we are suffering from a long list of health problems and diseases.

The more I've learnt about human evolution, the more I worry about what the future holds for all of

RIGHT *The Accumulator™ comes with access to an online community who will be taking part with you.*

us if we continue on this path. This book is my response to the need to change. I want you to discover how to move again, and to move in a way that your body wants you to. You may already go to a gym, but are you really pushing your body in the right direction to make it work to its best potential and therefore give you the best out of life? I also want you to consider how you eat and to challenge your relationship with food. Do you put food in your mouth that will work to make you healthy and strong, or that can potentially lead to sickness and therefore make you weak?

Many exercise plans, workout books and fitness DVDs on the market assume we are capable of going from zero to hero at the drop of a hat. We are all so fired up that we are ready to get up and go. We want to work out and work out hard. What often happens next, however, is that many of us find the experience to be so far out of our comfort zone that we give up very quickly and order a pizza.

The Accumulator™ is different. Whatever your current activity level and weight, I believe you will get something from this book. If you're on the first rung of the ladder to health and fitness, this book will get you to the top, one step at a time, day by day. If you already love the gym and consider yourself to have a good level of fitness, this book will challenge the way you think and make you see exercise in a new way for ever. It even comes with access to an online community who will be taking part with you, together with a library of resources to help you along the way.

The information and exercises in The Accumulator™ plan are designed for anyone aged between 18 and 65 with no medical conditions or physical restrictions that may hinder their ability to exercise safely. I also assume that you have no special dietary requirements, intolerances or allergies.

When using this book, you need to be aware of your personal physical health. In order to avoid injury or health problems, you should check with your doctor before beginning any fitness regime and be aware that you follow health, fitness and exercise advice at your own risk.

cigarettes and alcohol

I'll admit I used to smoke 20 plus per day and drink regularly but giving both up were amongst my wisest decisions. Alcohol is a subject I will touch on a little later in the book but if you do drink alcohol excessively or smoke, these can both clearly have a detrimental effect on your overall health and therefore the results you get from following the advice in this book.

So now is the time to discover where this all came from, learn how it all works and then we're off. Start on Day 1 and don't look back. By the time you've followed everything in this book it should look well-loved; the spine should be broken, some of the pages will be folded and torn, there will even be the odd sweat stain. That's fine – I want you to use and abuse this book.

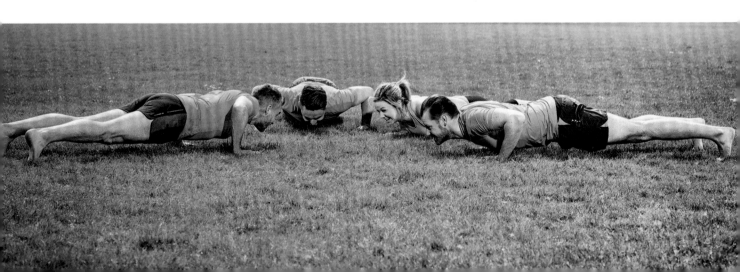

About me

I was reminiscing recently about my childhood with my mum. She told me how she is constantly amazed that I have ended up where I am now, doing what I do, when I was so negative about everything related to fitness as a child.

When I was growing up, I was overweight and inactive. I guess if I were young now I would be among the increasing number of children across the globe classed as obese. My diet was a carb-heavy horror story after I insisted on giving up meat as a 5-year-old and my mother struggled to feed me anything that was remotely healthy. The effect of this was weight gain and my total lack of interest in anything that brought about even the mildest of sweats.

Physical Education (PE) classes were a real battle for me, both physically and emotionally. I was always last, nobody would pick me for their team, and I felt humiliated as I had no aptitude or strength to have even a small hope of being average at anything. As a result, I hated exercise in all of its forms.

If I had been successful at winding my mum around my little finger (which was often) I would hand my teacher notes excusing me from participating in physical education classes. Especially if cross-country running was on the agenda.

Now health and fitness is such a major part of my life, I often find myself looking back on those days of cross-country runs, muddy knees and red faces. I have discovered a newfound respect for my old PE teacher and understand how hard he must have worked to try and motivate me and those like me.

Sadly, when I left school things went from bad to worse. Puberty had addressed issues regarding my shape to some

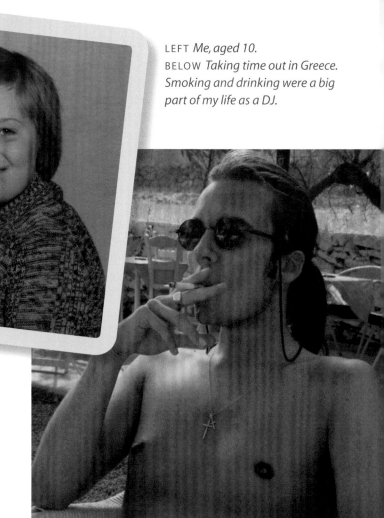

LEFT *Me, aged 10.*
BELOW *Taking time out in Greece. Smoking and drinking were a big part of my life as a DJ.*

degree, but as a young adult I continued to do as little exercise as possible and found comfort in cigarettes, alcohol and fast food. This fitted in nicely with my lifestyle as a DJ working in local clubs and eventually as a host on regional radio breakfast shows. I was a ticking time bomb. Many other guys in my situation may well have reached their forties or fifties before receiving some kind of wake-up call, but thankfully I got mine when I was only 30.

This catalyst for change was diagnosed as a disc herniation. Essentially, one of my intervertebral discs had burst, leaving me with intense pain in the lower regions of my back and down my legs. I had had an inkling that something was up for months before but had decided to ignore it and carry on regardless, coping as best I could with an increasingly large helping of painkillers. The tipping point came one morning when I found I could barely move. I can still clearly recall being fed by my wife Bridget while I was lying on the floor, just before my doctor came and insisted I should be in hospital. Bridget told me that I had to be injected with morphine into my hip before I was lifted into the ambulance. Thus began a long stretch in hospital, followed by many months of intensive physiotherapy before I could fully return to work.

It was one person, however, rather than the injury itself, who finally opened my eyes, saved my back and changed my life. That person was the physiotherapist assigned to work with me, who helped me build strength in my core to protect what is now a permanent weakness in my back. She taught me about the amazing group of muscles around my waist, and showed me what they are for and how to use them to protect my spine and save me from any more nights sleeping on the living room floor.

Thanks to my physio I suddenly realised that my muscular system played a far greater role in my body's functioning than just enabling me to compete against others. It was there to help me live my life in comfort, move with confidence and become fitter and stronger.

Curious to learn more, I read up on the subject and spent increasingly more time in my local gym. Eventually I ditched the beer, cigarettes and the bad diet. I had finally discovered a competition I could win, one in which I could challenge myself rather than struggling to compete against an opponent or a team. I quit my radio career and went back to school to learn everything I could about the body, and how I could help others to look after theirs better and be healthy for as long as possible.

Fifteen years on, and apart from the occasional twinge I am pain free, and in the best shape of my life. I now find myself at the helm of two fitness companies, contributing regular articles to fitness magazines and writing this book. I specialise in teaching functional exercise and barefoot running and have helped to change the lives of hundreds of people. There's nothing that satisfies me more than watching someone else's lightbulb go on as they overcome an injury or simply wake up to the many benefits that come with being fitter and healthier. But there are only so many hours in a day and I could only help a few people at a time; I wanted to share my discovery with lots of people at once.

I started posting month-long challenges on social media. Can you run 50km in a month? Can you build up to doing a 4-minute plank? Gradually, I accumulated an active community of participants who were hungry for whatever I could dream up next. So in my quest to fix people as I have fixed myself I developed The Accumulator™: a system that will help to change the habits that are causing many of today's health problems. At the same time, it deals with the two biggest excuses people have for not doing anything about their health: a lack of time and a lack of money.

BELOW *It was during a Sunday morning run through the fields near my home that the Accumulator™ was born.*

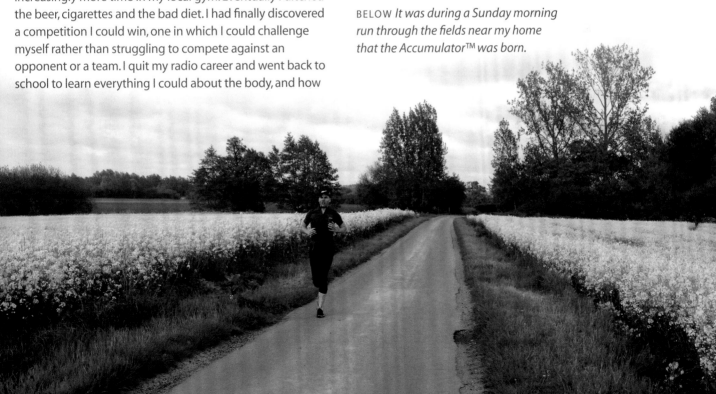

Creating the drive to succeed

YOU HAVE ALREADY TAKEN THE FIRST STEP TO BECOMING A FITTER, HEALTHIER AND BETTER VERSION OF YOURSELF BECAUSE YOU HAVE BOUGHT THIS BOOK. BEFORE YOU HAD IT YOU WERE ALREADY THINKING ABOUT DOING SOMETHING ABOUT YOUR STATE OF HEALTH AND YOU TOOK ACTION. NOW, WHILE THAT DESERVES A PAT ON THE BACK, IT'S ONLY THE BEGINNING. YOU'VE BOUGHT THE CAR AND YOU'VE GOT IN, NOW IT'S TIME TO START THE ENGINE AND *DRIVE*.

I've used the word 'drive' because that's the thing that will get you to the back page of this book having done everything it suggests. Your drive is your innate, biologically determined urge to attain a goal or satisfy a need. If you don't maintain it, you won't reach your destination. I want to tell you a little bit more about why your drive is so important and the amazing things you can achieve if you have lots of it.

BELOW *Your drive is your inate urge to attain a goal.*

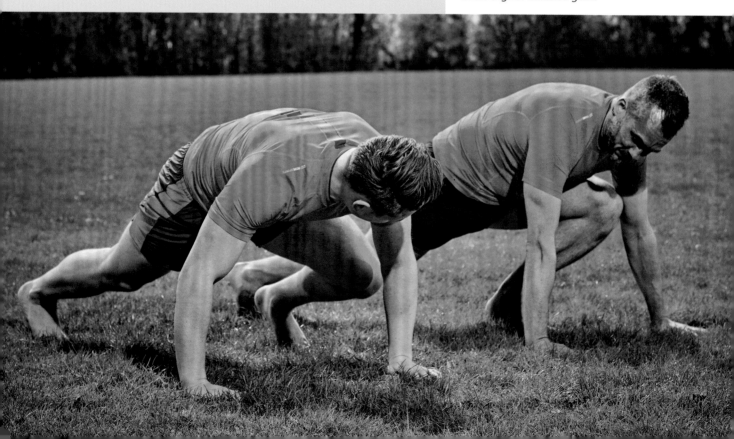

Believe you can do it

I often tell a story to my clients about Arnold Schwarzenegger. When he was around 20 years old, he spent some time staying with bodybuilder and movie star Reg Park in South Africa. When Reg asked him about his ambitions, the story goes that Arnold showed him a piece of paper with all his goals written on it. He wanted to win Mr Universe several times, as Reg had done. Then he wanted to become a movie star, a billionaire and go into politics. We all know what happened next. I have great admiration for Arnold. Not because of his bodybuilding accolades, his films or his politics but because of his belief in himself. Because of his drive. Here's a guy who grew up in a small farming community in Austria with no money and very few prospects, yet he believed he was going to achieve all these things, and he did.

When I decide to do something, no matter how big or small, I know right from the outset that I'm going to succeed. Let me share with you two methods I use that will help you achieve everything you set your mind to and to kick-start your own engine.

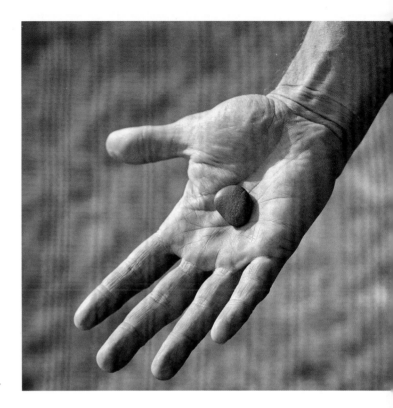

ABOVE *My gratitude stone.*

MAKE A LIST

Every year on my birthday I list three things I am going to achieve in the coming 12 months. I put that list on my office noticeboard, so that when I sit at my computer it's right in front of my face as a constant reminder of what I want to do. I actually don't need it written down at all, but in the moments when I lose my drive that list can pull me back on the road. Many people make New Year's resolutions and I guess what I do is the same – I just pick a different date on which to make them. Your list could be positioned anywhere or in multiple places. If the goals are really important to you, after a few weeks you probably won't need your list at all – you will be able to recall your aims instantly.

GET STONED

Do you have a friend who can find good in everything, or take a really bad situation and flip it on its head? Aren't those types of people great to be around? Do you find yourself saying 'I wish I could be like that'? Well, you can. It just takes practice.

Every day I revel in all that is positive in my life. It may sound stupid, but many of us just let the good things pass us by and never appreciate how lucky we really are. Even if it seems like you're at rock bottom, you're not. I have a small stone in my pocket that I have carried with me everywhere since my daughter gave it to me on our favourite beach when she was 4 years old. Nobody else would find that stone particularly special, but each time I reach into my pocket and feel it it reminds me of my daughter and all the other good things I have in my life.

You can do the same thing. Pick something that has a positive association, that reminds you of a time when

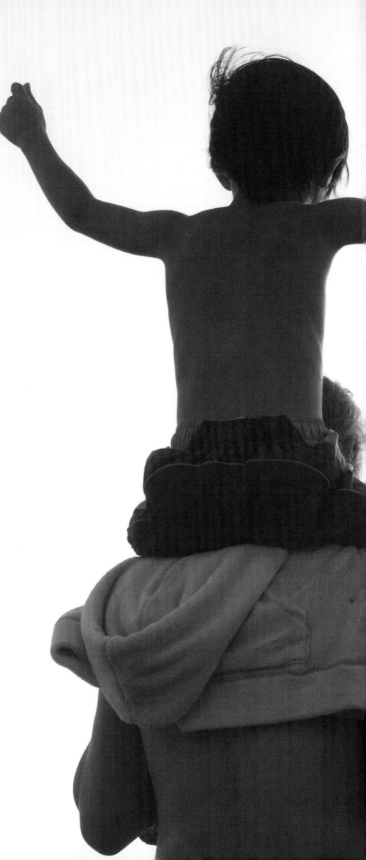

you were happy or of someone you love. Your 'stone' will help you be positive because it will jerk you back into that good state of mind whenever you look at it or touch it, and maintain your positive drive.

What's your destination?

It doesn't matter if you want to lose weight, run a marathon, get a six-pack or even do your first push-up. Whatever your goal, if you have a positive frame of mind and plenty of drive, it will happen. If you start your workout thinking 'I really don't want to do this, I'm not going to do well today', you will begin to lose your drive very quickly. However, if you approach it thinking 'I'm going to work hard, think about why I'm doing it and be grateful that I can do it at all' then you'll find the motivation you need and head to the shower feeling great about yourself.

Before you read any further, find a piece of paper. Now write down one thing you want more than anything else. We know you want to improve your fitness or you wouldn't be reading this, but really nail it down to specifics. Why do you want to get fitter? What part of your life do you want to improve by becoming fitter? Do you want to improve the way you look? Do you want to be able to play with your kids without getting out of breath? Do you want to be able to control a supermarket trolley?

Digging a little deeper might take longer and you might even write down a few things before you find the real reason why you want to improve your fitness, but that's OK. Be totally honest with yourself – nobody else has to see what you've written down.

Let's go back to the car for a few minutes. The engine is running and we're now dealing with your destination. What would you do if you were actually in a real car about to go on a journey? You'd know where you were going right down to the postcode and the door number wouldn't you? You wouldn't just drive to a city and then hope you got lucky finding the right place; you'd plan. You'd know exactly where your destination was.

Focusing on what you want in this way is vital to maintaining your drive. The more specific you can make your goal, the more you will move heaven and earth to make sure you achieve it because you can visualise it. Have you ever booked a holiday and pictured how the place will look when you get there? What it will feel like lying on the beach or how delicious the food will taste? Have you ever wanted something so much that you imagine what it would feel like to already have it?

I remember when I was a child I had a friend called Tony. He had all the latest toys in his bedroom. The thing with Tony, however, was that even though he had all this stuff, he didn't appreciate any of it. He didn't really value it because he didn't earn it. He wasn't grateful for it because he didn't really want it in the first place.

Think of all the things you've done in your own life that you have really been proud of. Did you work for them or did they just fall into your lap? Did they result from hard work or did they come easily? The things we really appreciate and cherish are usually the outcome of effort, determination and … here it comes … wait for it … drive.

By now you should have something really specific written down on your piece of paper and you may be really fired up to achieve it. It's no longer 'I want to be fitter', it's 'I want to be able to run for a bus' or 'I want to be able to fit into those jeans I've had my eye on'.

Now here's another question: *when* do you want it? Let's get back into your car again for a second. You're in the driving seat, the engine's on and you now know exactly where you're going. You can see

your destination in your mind's eye. You may even know what colour the front door is (mine is red by the way). Now, when do you want to arrive? Fixing an end date by which you aim to achieve your goal will help you to maintain your drive because you can have the finish line in your sights from the very beginning.

When deciding upon a date, think about where you are right now. If you've been unfit and unhealthy for 20 years, you're not going to change in 20 days. If it's taken you two years to gain 2 stones in weight, you won't lose it in two months. However, if you're already active but just want to take it up a notch, learn some new skills and try something different, that's a goal you can achieve in a much shorter length of time. The important thing to bear in mind is the longer you have to spend on the journey, the more driving you'll have to do, but you'll always be getting closer to the destination. Just imagine you have to travel to the other side of the world. The chances are you won't make your journey in one go. You might even consider breaking the trip up to make it easier to cope with, scheduling a stop-off or two along the way. Guess what? The same applies here. If you've decided it's going to take you two years to get what you really want, you know it's going to be a long journey – so why not break it up into a series of smaller goals? Schedule a few stop-offs?

Now, here's where this plan really helps. The Accumulator™ can be one of those smaller goals. The mission is to complete the whole plan, and you will be able to do this in just 30 days. Doing it represents the first step on a really exciting new path and, having proved to yourself that you can achieve one leg of the journey, it should give you the confidence to go the distance.

Why make the change?

Why do I exercise and eat good food? Because I want to be able to walk my daughter down the aisle, dance with her on her wedding day and play with her children. Not because I want to look good in jeans and a T-shirt.

Learning to move

Fit for life

Prior to the advent of modern technology we would use our bodies (and our brains) to help us survive. We were expert hunters and regularly ran for many miles to chase animals that we could eat. We then developed basic tools to help us gather food, build homes and eventually to grow our own crops. Back then, living was all the exercise we needed. Even as recently as a century ago people did more exercise just to survive than we do now. The car was a still a luxury and many of us relied on our feet, a pushbike, or a horse if we were lucky and could afford one. Just imagine yourself doing something as ordinary as the weekly food shop a hundred years ago.

A S A RACE, WE'VE BECOME A LITTLE TOO CLEVER FOR OUR OWN GOOD. IN AN ATTEMPT TO MAKE OUR LIVES MORE CONVENIENT AND MORE COMFORTABLE WE HAVE BECOME FAR LESS ACTIVE AND THEREBY STARTED TO DAMAGE OUR OWN HEALTH AND OUR FITNESS. AS A RESULT WE ARE NOW A LONG WAY FROM THE PHYSICALLY STRONGER AND MORE CAPABLE SPECIES THAT MADE US SO SUCCESSFUL IN THE FIRST PLACE.

Our bodies are designed to move. Our evolutionary success is in part thanks to our ability to walk, run, lift, twist, crawl, push, pull and move in many different ways with skill. When you think about it, we are pretty amazing. Now, however, exercise is at best regarded as a hobby in Western culture. When you consider how far the evolutionary process has brought us to date, it makes you wonder what we will evolve into in another thousand years.

Exercise in any form is important: I consider it just as important as eating. You may well survive for longer without exercise than without food, but if you omit it altogether, your body will not be able to function properly and in the long term you'll be in trouble. So if it is such a vital thing for our health what exercise should you do? The answer is simple: exercise should be something that makes you better at everything you do, better at *living*. You should work out to improve your quality of life. However, many people approach fitness in the wrong way and think

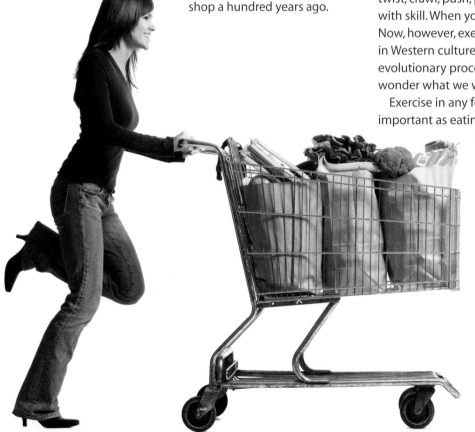

about how they look first and how they function second. If you exercise to achieve a better quality of life, you will end up looking better as a result. This won't necessarily work the other way around, however, and focusing foremost on your appearance can result in a failure to improve fitness, or even injury.

I often find myself using a classic exercise such as a bicep curl as a good example of this upside-down approach to fitness. In one of the gyms I regularly visit there is a free-weights section facing a floor-to-ceiling mirror. Regularly on a Friday afternoon a group of young men arrive to work on their biceps. They spend an hour finding as many different ways as they can to bend their arms at the elbow and lift weight up to their shoulders while admiring their bulging muscles in the mirror. For achieving bigger biceps, there's no doubt that this can be a very effective approach, but think about this for a second. What function does that exercise serve? Where else, apart from in a gym, do you see anyone moving in that way? Bending the elbow with resistance forms a part of many other movements but we never do it in isolation.

Whether you want to become better at a chosen sport or simply just to function well in everyday life, exercise should be a tool that will help to make it possible. Many people approach exercise one muscle or one joint at a time, but our muscular system is just that, a system, with so many different muscles that are designed to work together.

Think of all the movements you make every day that involve a degree of strength. How about something like pushing and controlling a heavy supermarket trolley or cart. That's a nightmare isn't it? You want to go one way and your trolley wants to go the other. Hit a pothole in the car park and you're close to disaster as you visualise all your groceries spilling out over the floor. That journey to your car that you take for granted involves you using your thighs, your bum, many of the muscles in your core, your back and your shoulders – all at once. Then you get to the car, open the boot or trunk and lift heavy bags out of the trolley and into your car while fighting to prevent the trolley from wandering off towards the car next to you. Back, hips and bum, core, shoulders, arms (including biceps) and even your chest all work together to make this happen. Performing such simple, banal movements as these is actually one of

the most common ways for people to suffer injuries, so it is important you are fit for life.

Here's a really good example of why it's important you do the right type of exercise. A woman I met said she had been suffering with back problems for some time and was seeing an osteopath. Her osteopath advised her to do a plank exercise to strengthen her core. The plank is a stationary exercise that requires you to support yourself close to the floor by holding your body up using your feet and

ABOVE *The human body is designed to move.*

forearms. She told me she was getting really good at the plank and could hold it for several minutes. However, every time she tried to load or unload the dishwasher she still suffered from terrible back pain. While the plank is a great exercise for helping to increase core strength, it wasn't of any practical use here. To her it was like becoming an expert swimmer when she needed to run a marathon.

So, let's go back to my original question. What exercises should you do? The answer is: ones that help you to do everything you want to do. I have designed The Accumulator™ to be useful. It's filled with exercises and movements that will help you to function better when you're not working out. I have always believed in this principle as a coach. It doesn't matter if I'm training a runner, a tennis player or someone who simply wants to be able to dig the garden without getting backache. All I'm doing is helping that person to live a better life and that's really all most people want to achieve. When we get to the exercise plan later in this book I will explain how each exercise can help you in your everyday life.

Why Accumulate?

SO WE ALREADY KNOW THAT BODYWEIGHT EXERCISE IS ONE OF THE MOST EFFECTIVE FORMS OUT THERE. THE BENEFITS YOU CAN GAIN FROM A BODYWEIGHT WORKOUT, AND IN PARTICULAR THE ACCUMULATOR™, ARE HUGE. IN THIS CHAPTER I'LL EXPLAIN HOW THE ACCUMULATOR™ CAN BENEFIT YOU.

I could easily sit here and tell you that I designed The Accumulator™ knowing in advance exactly how it would work and what the benefits would be. But I'm going to be honest. Many of the pluses to be gained from using this model didn't actually occur to me until I'd been testing out The Accumulator™ for some months. Don't get me wrong – I realised it was good from the start and I knew there were plenty of boxes I fully intended to tick when I designed it. However, some of the more subtle advantages from working in this way didn't really materialise until I started seeing it all work for the many people who have taken part.

before I start...

I'd just like to point out that I'm going to make the assumption that you do very little or no regular exercise at present. If fitness is already a part of your life and you're reading this book because you want to try something different, that's great – I am certain you will benefit from this plan too. There are already many people who combine The Accumulator™ with other forms of exercise and gain an awful lot from it, and this chapter will help you to understand just how versatile The Accumulator™ really is.

aspect, because if you persistently move with bad form you will run the risk of becoming injured, if not straight away, then perhaps at some point down the line. This is something I'm particularly passionate about, as I've helped and continue to help many people who have been exercising for years but doing things incorrectly. It's not until they start to move properly that the right muscles activate, niggling injuries go away and they feel more confident, get stronger and become fitter than they were before. It's not their fault that they got it wrong. In fact it's human nature to find short cuts, but not all quick routes are beneficial. For example, when I was learning to drive, I developed a habit of turning the steering wheel with the palm of one open hand. It's really lazy and actually a dangerous way to turn a corner – something my driving instructor reminded me of regularly – but many years after passing my driving test I find myself

Learn to move

First and foremost, The Accumulator™ helps you to learn how to exercise properly. This is a really important doing it from time to time. I know it's wrong, I can hear my driving instructor in my head telling me it's wrong, yet I still do it because it's just easier than threading the steering wheel through my hands.

The same reversion to easy but bad habits can apply to exercise, which is why it's important to go back to basics so you can learn the correct way to move. Right at the start of The Accumulator™ I will show you some fundamental body movements. Even if you think you can do them properly, there's a fairly big chance that you will benefit from revisiting them in their most simple form. Due to the structured nature of The Accumulator™ you will have to do these exercises every single day (apart from on rest days). Repeating the movements like this works in two different ways: first, you will become better at performing them as the month progresses; second, they will grow increasingly harder to perform because of the accumulating workout that will be performed before you get to them. At the start of the month the moves will be the majority of the workout and you'll come at them fresh, but by the end of the month your muscles will be tired when you do them.

RIGHT *From the start of The Accumulator™ I will show you some fundamental body movements.*

In addition, you'll notice that these basic movements will pop up again later on in the month as an accompaniment to something else, which will make doing them more of a challenge.

Many of the actions in The Accumulator™ are big ones. I believe in using as much of your body as possible at the same time. Not only because this is how we move anyway (think about all the muscles you use to throw a ball, for instance), but because the more muscles you activate the more energy you need to do it, and the more energy you need, the more you expend.

Take the time

There are many popular excuses when it comes to exercise and The Accumulator™ confounds all of them. The most common one I've heard is 'I don't have the time'. You may have even heard yourself say it. I'm sorry to burst your bubble but you actually do have the time for everything. When I

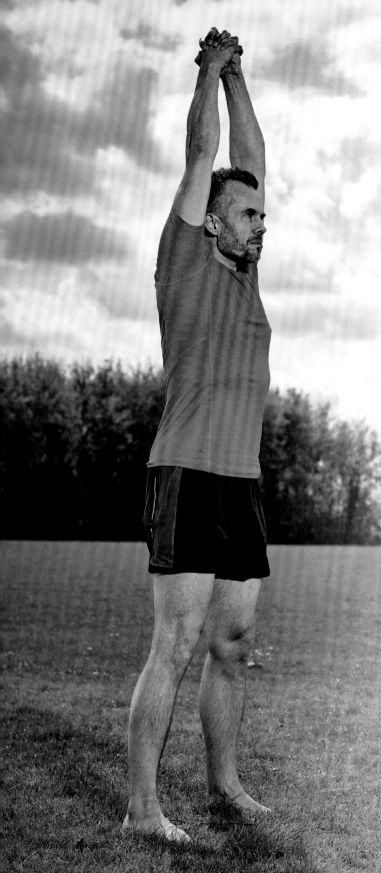

hear the phrase 'I don't have time' what I actually hear is 'this is not important to me'.

The vast majority of us choose what we do with our day; most things you do are a direct result of a choice you made at some point (there are some exceptions to this rule I know, but on the whole you'll find it holds true). If you don't find time for exercise you have made this choice: you have decided it is not a priority for you. However, we all know what happens when we don't move our bodies – they stop functioning as they should. Well, your priorities are about to change. You've obviously already decided that exercise needs to become a bigger part of your life, even if you are busy, because you've bought my book (or someone bought it for you). My job is to help you overcome the urge to just sit down at the end of the day and instead to use the time to benefit your whole life. I am going to tell you right now how to re-wire your brain and fiddle about with all those connections in there so you become hard-wired to love exercise.

On the first day of The Accumulator™ all I want you to do is exercise for 40 seconds. That's it. That's less time than it takes to boil the kettle. In fact you can do day one while you boil the kettle. By the end of Week 1 the total time you'll be exercising for is just four minutes. As you enter the second week, something will start to happen. As long as you follow the plan, you'll notice your muscles will start to react, your cardiovascular system will become challenged. Most importantly, chemicals will be released by your body that interact with receptors in your brain to make you think you're actually having a good time. Your body is designed to make exercise feel good because exercise is important to the survival of the human race. Sex and eating feel good because the same chemical process is going on in your brain when we do it, for the same reason.

The point I'm making here is this: exercise makes you feel good when you do it and the benefits it produces make you feel even better. If you're not already exercising on a regular basis, or are doing the wrong kind of exercise, you probably won't have felt that high before. So it's no wonder you don't want to do it. By taking baby steps into The Accumulator™, your body will begin to feel the positive effects and it will start to become a habit, and then a priority. Suddenly you will have time to do it because you will make time to do it.

Take your gym with you

In addition to not taking long to do, The Accumulator™ can be done anywhere, making it incredibly time-efficient. Many people think doing exercise involves taking a huge chunk out of your day – driving to a gym, getting ready, queuing for equipment, showering and driving home. The truth is, working out doesn't have to take long at all. With The Accumulator™ you don't need to go anywhere, you don't need loads of space and you don't need to invest in lots of expensive equipment. Wherever you are, whether at home or on holiday, you have your gym with you. You are your gym.

Many people who have taken part in The Accumulator™ have demonstrated just how practical it really is. One particular lady who comes to mind is Gillian. She is fortunate enough to have sufficient resources to be able to enjoy her retirement by going on lots of holidays and having many adventures. She has been doing The Accumulator™ non-stop since I launched it and has sent me numerous pictures from all over the world of her doing her workouts in various locations. You can see some of these in the back of this book.

The Accumulator™ has also appealed to many mothers in the past. If you've ever had young children, you will understand how difficult it is to find any time at all for yourself. One young mum told me how she manages to fit her workout in at a moment's notice. When her daughter has an afternoon sleep or is happy playing, she uses the time to exercise. She doesn't have to arrange childminding, which she would require to go to the gym, and she doesn't have to prepare in advance; if an opportunity to work out arises, she seizes it.

BELOW *The Accumulator™ is ideal for those with little ones to look after.*

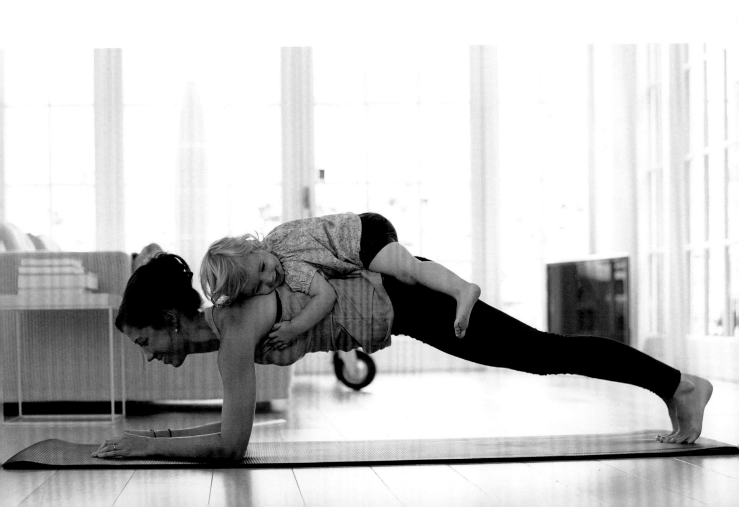

Eating right for life

BEFORE YOU READ ON I WANT YOU TO KNOW THIS IS NOT A CHAPTER ABOUT WEIGHT LOSS. IT'S NOT EVEN A BOOK ABOUT WEIGHT LOSS. EVEN THOUGH YOUR WEIGHT MAY CHANGE AS A RESULT OF DOING EVERYTHING IN THIS BOOK, IT ALSO MAY NOT. THE ACCUMULATOR™ IS ABOUT MUCH MORE THAN THIS – THERE IS A MUCH BIGGER PICTURE.

I WANT THIS BOOK TO HELP TRANSFORM YOU INTO THE BEST POSSIBLE VERSION OF YOURSELF BY BECOMING BETTER AT MOVING THE WAY YOUR BODY WANTS YOU TO. I ALSO WANT TO INSPIRE YOU TO PUT THE BEST FOOD INTO YOUR BODY AND BECOME THE HEALTHIEST, FITTEST PERSON YOU CAN BE.

LEFT *The scales won't tell you everything you need to know.*

Let's just deal with those two words for a second: weight loss. What do they really mean? The world is struggling with a massive health problem and a large percentage of the population is becoming overweight or obese. Many of us eat a terrible diet packed with man-made processed foods and added sugar. We also don't move anywhere near enough to keep our bodies healthy. Now, these lifestyle changes may be making us fatter and less healthy, but is 'losing weight' really the solution?

Take a look at yourself in the mirror. What do you see? You are a collection of organs, bones, muscle and fat. All these ingredients weigh something and collectively they make up the number you see when you step on a weighing scale. The only person who sees that number is you (and perhaps your doctor). Your family, friends and everyone you meet just see you and what shape you are. In order to live a healthier life, move better and change your reflection you may not need to change your weight at all. You just need to change the relative quantities of some of your component parts and this will change your silhouette.

So which of your constituent parts should you try to change?

1

INTERNAL ORGANS Unless you have some of these removed through surgery or you have some form of medical condition, your organs are unlikely to change that much in terms of size and weight (although your whole body composition, including organ size, can change as you get older).

2

BONES AND CONNECTIVE TISSUE (LIGAMENTS AND TENDONS) Making these stronger and therefore heavier is extremely beneficial, helping to prevent health issues such as osteoporosis and making them less likely to break. With the right nutrition and regular exercise you can make this happen.

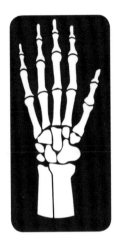

3

MUSCLES The size and weight of your muscle mass has a huge impact on your shape. This is something I'll come on to in more detail later but, in a nutshell, you want more of the stuff. First, more muscle makes you stronger and therefore more able to do things. Second, the more muscle you have, the more fuel your body needs to keep that muscle tissue in tip-top condition. So I think we can agree that you really don't want to make your muscles smaller and lighter.

4

FAT Your body does need some of it, but many people have much more than is necessary and this is a major problem. Ultimately, it's too much fat that can lead to a multitude of life-threatening illnesses and I think most people would agree that fat spilling over jeans is not a great thing to see in the mirror. So, body fat is the stuff you want to lose.

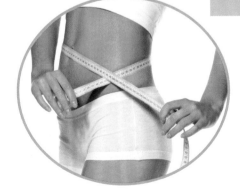

As you can see, you actually want more of some of the constituent parts that make up your body – it's only fat that you want less of. So why do we place so much importance on the number on the scales when it doesn't really tell us what we need to know? Many people become obsessed with that figure and I've had to wean people off their scale addiction in the past because they want to step on them once every day or sometimes even more frequently. If you've ever been to a slimming club, the chances are your progress has been measured on a set of scales and you've found that some weeks you did better than others. The problem with measuring your weight on a regular basis is that it naturally fluctuates. The time of day, what you have eaten, when you last visited the bathroom, even the balance of your hormones and how much sleep you've had can have an effect on your overall weight. So stepping on the scales daily won't necessarily show you the positive impact exercise and diet can have on your body – on the way it looks and moves.

Can you now see why it's more important to focus on changing your shape rather than your weight? In order to do this, you need to focus on altering your body's composition. Now, if you have a lot of body fat to lose, the number on the scales will probably become smaller when you do The Accumulator™ plan. For many of us, however, it may not change too much at all. If you rely on the weighing scales and nothing else as a gauge by which you measure your success, the result of The Accumulator™ as a 'weight-loss' plan will probably be more than a little disappointing. This doesn't mean you have failed. You're simply measuring the wrong thing.

I mentioned muscle mass a little earlier and the dramatic effect it can have on your shape. Muscle is important because not only does it make you stronger and more capable, but it also requires energy to make it work and keep it healthy. The more of it you have, the more energy you will need to stop it wasting away. That in turn means that if you're eating the right food your body will need to

BELOW *Body weight exercises help increase muscle mass.*

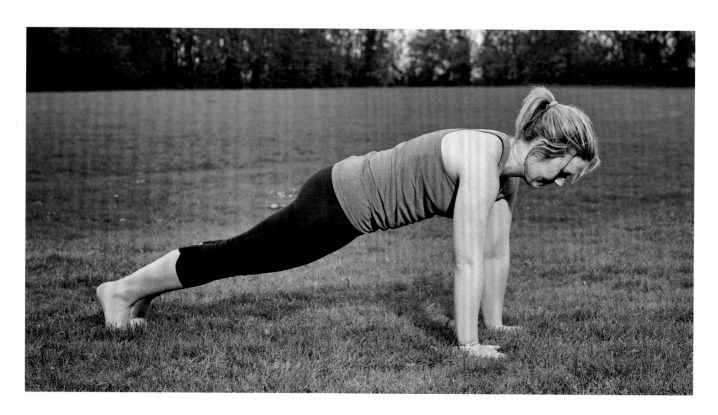

dip into your fat stores more often in order to keep your muscles working properly.

An increase in muscle mass is an essential element when it comes to improving your health and fitness and this goes for both men and women. Many females shy away from any form of resistance exercise because they believe they will end up looking too muscular and bulky. This is simply not true, as women can't grow muscle tissue in the same way as men, since they have a much lower level of testosterone. In fact, men have around eight times more testosterone than women and this is partly why women look like women and not like men. Many women (and men) will refer to a 'toned' appearance when describing how they want to look. A toned body is simply one with a greater muscle mass and a lower fat mass. If this is how you visualise the ideal version of yourself, you may already have a bigger muscle mass on your shopping list and not even realise it.

Measuring up

Now that we've established you don't really need the scales to determine any changes in your body, how can you best measure your success? Many years ago, when I was a fledgling personal trainer, I started spending more time in gyms, I learned much more about how my body works, my diet improved and I just placed more importance on looking healthy. After all, who wants to hire a trainer who looks like they don't take their own advice? I remember being invited to the wedding of one of my former colleagues. There were lots of people present who I hadn't seen for a couple of years and nearly all of them asked if I had lost weight. In fact, I had actually gained weight as my muscle mass had gone up and my body fat had gone down, along with the size of my clothes. It just looked like I had lost weight. So, if the biggest change is actually reflected in your appearance, then that's exactly what you should monitor.

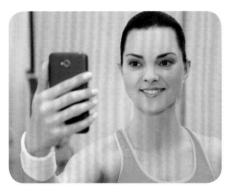

TAKE A PHOTO This is a really powerful way to measure your success. It's best to ask a friend to help, but a selfie in the mirror will do. Strip down to your underwear (or get naked if you really want to, just make sure you keep the evidence to yourself). Take two photos, one face on and one in profile.

TAKE SOME MEASUREMENTS You will see your shape change in the mirror, and you'll notice it in your clothes too. So grab a tape measure. Start around your waist; make sure the tape is level and measure at the level of your belly button. This will ensure that you measure in exactly the same place next time. Next, go to your thighs and measure these at the widest point of your hips. Finally measure around your chest using your nipples as a guide. These are the three areas where you are likely to see the biggest changes in your shape because these are the places where our bodies tend to lay down the most fat.

PICK OUT SOME CLOTHES This is a really powerful gauge. If your shape has changed as you have aged, you may still have something in your wardrobe that you can no longer fit into. Take it out and try it on. Take a photo of yourself wearing it (or maybe trying to). That item of clothing has now not only become your measure of success, but it's also a very good motivating tool.

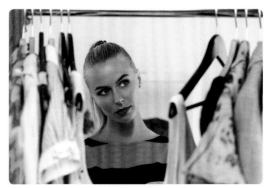

Eating right for life

A diet is simply the collective term for all the things you eat and drink, good or bad. It is not a six-week miracle plan, it's not a pull-out from a magazine and it's definitely not a meal replacement drink. It is something you do for ever. One of my favourite phrases is, 'any temporary change will only give you temporary results' and that's very true when it comes to your diet. If you only change it for a few weeks or months you will not see permanent results. Permanent change comes from *making* permanent change.

So, to be successful at transforming your diet from a bad one to a good one and ultimately becoming the healthiest you can be, the only thing you need to do is change what you eat – and never look back. Many of the food choices we make on a day-to-day basis are just habits. Everyone has these, and some are better than others. The Accumulator™ works to help you to make good choices. Here's a list of common bad eating habits – see how many of these you recognise:

- The need to clear your plate.
- Eating something sweet after each meal.
- Buying cakes to celebrate someone's birthday.
- Running out of time and resorting to fast food or takeaways.
- Snacking on junk food in front of the TV or at the movies.
- Skipping breakfast.
- Eating when you're sad, stressed or around a period.
- Eating in the car or on the go.
- Rushing your food.

BELOW *Include plenty of fresh fruit and vegetables in your meals.*

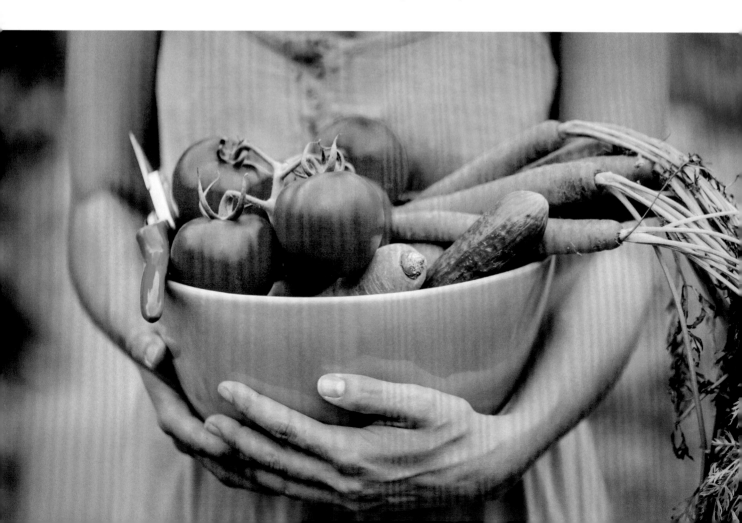

There are many things that should be considered when it comes to eating a healthy diet. I've always found that if you understand something, you can implement it far more effectively. Whenever I talk to someone about their diet I always make sure they comprehend my simple laws of food so they know what food really is and how our bodies use it. Being armed with a basic knowledge of nutrition will help you to *want* to make the right food choices, but it may not necessarily make your diet change in the long term. In order to do this, you will need to break some bad food-related habits.

The laws of food

Before we head into your eating plan I want you to understand the laws of food. These are my nuggets of knowledge that will help you to turn your bad habits into good ones. I'm going to keep this simple. There are many books on nutrition out there that go into the subject in depth but, while they are fascinating, unless you have an understanding of the fundamentals they can be a little daunting and confusing, and the whole thing may feel too much like hard work. But it really doesn't need to be. If you manage to follow the following simple laws of food and do nothing else, your body will begin to thank you for it.

LAW 1: EAT FOOD AND ONLY FOOD

Not all food is actually food. This may seem like a stupid thing to say, but go to your local supermarket, look around and notice what they are selling more of, food or just products made from food. Many people survive on a diet made up of mainly food products and not real food. The difference between the two is simple but huge:

- **FOOD: EVERYTHING WE EAT OR DRINK THAT CAME FROM THE EARTH, ABOVE THE EARTH OR ON THE EARTH.**

- **FOOD PRODUCTS: EVERYTHING WE EAT OR DRINK THAT'S MAN-MADE USING ONLY SOME OF THE THINGS MENTIONED ABOVE.**

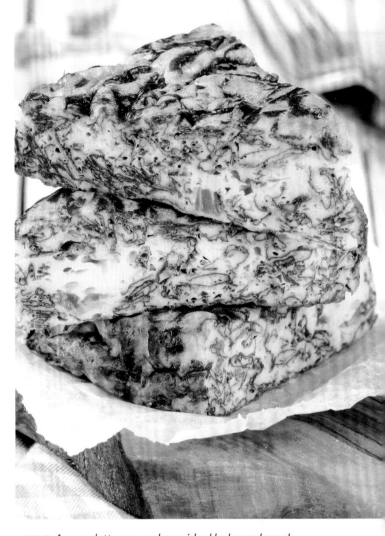

ABOVE *An omelette can make an ideal balanced meal.*

If you follow this law, a banana is food. An omelette made with spinach, onion and mushrooms is food. A loaf of bread containing preservatives, stabilisers and added vitamins is a food product. A frozen microwaveable lasagne containing thickeners, wheat starch, hydrolysed vegetable protein and niacin is a food product. All the information you require to make good food choices is right there on every single label – you just need to know what to look for. The best food is the stuff you can buy with no labels at all, but if there is a label then the fewer things there are in the ingredients list the better. If there is anything on that list you can't pronounce, walk away. It's almost certainly a food product.

LAW 2: UNDERSTAND WHAT'S IN YOUR FOOD

I'm not talking about the ingredients list here, but instead about macronutrients. These are the three main components of everything we eat and drink and they all do very important things inside us. All three are essential for health, which is why a diet that eliminates one of them is not going to lead to long-term health. It's pretty important that you know what they are and what they do.

CARBOHYDRATE = ENERGY

All carbohydrates are broken down inside us into sugars, which give us energy. Various types of carbohydrate break down at different rates and therefore give us different amounts of energy for certain periods of time. Imagine a scale from 1 to 100. At one end there are simple carbohydrates and at the other end are complex carbohydrates. This scale from simple to complex is often referred to as the glycaemic index (GI). The best way to explain how carbohydrates work is with the help of the bathtub metaphor.

The bathtub metaphor

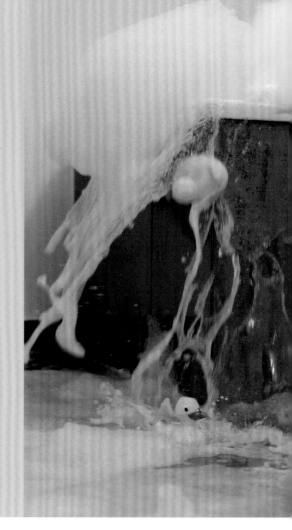

BATH NUMBER 1

Put in the plug and turn on the taps as far as they can go so the bath fills up very quickly. As soon as it is full, pull out the plug so the bath empties as quickly as possible. This is how simple (high-GI) carbohydrates work in your body. They are converted into energy very quickly and burn out very quickly and then you are hungry again (or the bath is empty).

BATH NUMBER 2

This time only turn on one tap so there's a very small trickle of water coming out and the bath takes a long time to fill. Before it becomes completely full, reach for the plug and just turn it slightly on to one side so a small amount of water can escape down the drain. This is similar to the effect complex (low-GI) carbohydrates have on your body. These are generally less calorie-dense so you have to eat a larger quantity to get the same amount of energy as you'd get from simple carbohydrates, which means you're less likely to eat too much in one sitting. Compare a baked potato to a small chocolate bar for instance. They both contain a similar number of calories but it will take you far longer to eat the potato. Your body has to work much harder to get at the sugar in a complex carbohydrate; therefore it will supply you with a slower, steady trickle of energy for longer.

Carbohydrate-rich foods for your shopping list:

- Green vegetables
- Root vegetables (don't include too many white potatoes; try sweet ones instead as they have a lower GI)
- Beans and pulses
- Wholegrain rice
- Quinoa
- Oats
- Fruit (but not fruit juice)
- Some wholewheat or granary bread.

BATH NUMBER 3

This time turn the taps on any way you like. Turn on one or two, fully on or trickling – it doesn't matter. Now put in the plug, block up the overflow outlet, get in and fall asleep. Eventually the bath will over-fill unless you pull out the plug and get rid of the water and you'll end up with puddles on the bathroom floor.

Imagine if you left it running for several days and the damage it would do. This is what happens when you don't burn the energy carbohydrates give you. With more sugar than you need your body begins to store it as fat or, even worse, it struggles to deal with the amount you're giving it and certain functions or organs start running into trouble. This is why carbohydrates get blamed for our weight problems. Our body needs some to function, but when we continually eat more than we need we become very good at storing fat and eventually deeper problems start to emerge.

Even if you only over-fill your bath by a little bit each day, you will still end up with accumulating puddles of water on the carpet. In my career as a fitness expert, I have analysed countless food diaries and I have never had to tell someone they are eating too little carbohydrate.

A FEW WORDS ABOUT BREAD

There is an argument that humans are not supposed to be eating bread at all and many of us are intolerant to wheat or gluten which means it can leave us feeling 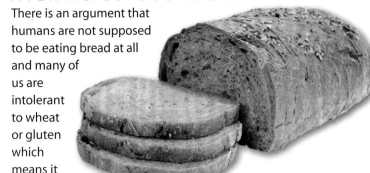 bloated or uncomfortable. Personally I eat very little bread for that reason and the only bread that doesn't disagree with me is the stuff I make myself. So while bread is on the list I would suggest you keep it to a minimum (occasionally rather than daily). I also suggest you stick to fresh wholegrain or granary bread from a baker (or the bakery counter). Bread should only contain basic ingredients and should begin to turn stale after a few days. Processed bread is very different and can live in your kitchen happily for much longer before going mouldy and not stale.

PROTEIN = BUILDING BLOCKS

We are made from protein. Our organs, hair, skin and muscles are made from the stuff, not to mention our DNA. All other animals are made from protein too. We can make some of our own protein inside us but we also need to eat some in order to keep our bodies healthy and repair any damage that may occur. In the same way that carbohydrates break down into sugar, protein breaks down into amino acids. There are 20 different types of amino acid and we have to eat food to obtain nine of them. If we want our muscles to get bigger, our connective tissue to become stronger and our body to function properly, we need protein. If you didn't eat any, your body would slowly break down your muscles to get what it needs.

Many people struggle with protein and simply don't eat enough of it. Because carbs are so readily available and form the basis of most processed foods we tend to over-eat these at the expense of protein and therefore we lack the right resources to build muscle. The big bonus with protein is it fills you up and keeps you feeling satisfied for a long time, much more so than carbohydrates. It's very difficult to over-eat protein for that reason, but it's very easy to binge on carbs. Have you ever snacked on chocolate or cookies until you felt sick? So have I. Ever done that with a chicken?

Protein-rich foods for your shopping list:
- Unprocessed meat and poultry (preferably organic)
- Sustainable fish and shellfish (salmon, white fish, mackerel, tuna)
- Dairy (unprocessed/full-fat)
- Organic eggs
- Nuts and seeds.

FAT = PROTECTION
OK, let's get something straight from the start. Fat is good. We need to eat fat because without it our body is in deep trouble. For starters, we require a small layer of fat to protect our internal organs from damage. We also need it to process some important vitamins (called fat-soluble vitamins), and we can use fat for energy. In fact, it's a very good source of energy but because we're eating too many carbohydrates it very rarely gets a look in.

It's also very unlikely that fat will make you fat. This is because, on its own, it's very hard to eat too much of it (combine it with carbs, though, and it's a monster – think doughnuts). There's a high likelihood that the majority of your body fat is as a result of over-eating carbohydrates and not from eating too much fat.

All fat is not equal though. There are two basic types: saturated and unsaturated. Until quite recently it was thought that a diet high in saturated fat was bad for us, but there is an increasing body of evidence that suggests this may not be the case and which questions the accuracy of some studies done in the past on dietary fat and its effect on our bodies. In the time between writing this book and you reading it the news on saturated fat will undoubtedly change so it's unfair for me to make any sweeping statements here. However, if your fat comes from unprocessed foods (see the foods in the shopping list), and you don't eat too much of it, you can't go far wrong. There is, however, a third kind of fat called trans-fat or hydrogenated fat. This is fat used in some processed foods that has been treated with hydrogen, which changes its structure and makes it very damaging to our health. Thankfully, this type isn't as abundant as it once was, and if you avoid processed food (see Law 1) you'll be fine.

A few words about eggs and chickens

Think about an egg for a second. In that shell is everything needed to make a chicken. It's a tiny bomb of goodness filled with protein, fats and a multitude of minerals and vitamins. However, what goes in the chicken comes out in the egg, so a chicken that's kept in a cage and not allowed to enjoy grass, seeds and the odd juicy worm is not going to produce an egg that's as nutritious as one that comes out of a chicken that can forage for those things, exercise and consume a diet free from antibiotics and pesticides.

If you want to enjoy the best eggs possible, get your own chickens. I know this isn't an option for everyone, but if you have the space for some, do it. I recently took the plunge and now have four. They are easy to look after, full of character and they give me the best-tasting eggs I have ever had. You will not want to buy an egg from a supermarket again … If you can't keep chickens, track down your nearest farm shop that does keep them and buy their eggs instead.

Fat-rich foods on for your shopping list:

- Coconut oil (for cooking)
- Olive oil (for dressing)
- Nuts
- Seeds
- Fish (see protein)
- Butter; dairy; avocados.

LAW 3: THINK QUALITY OVER QUANTITY

This is going to shock you, but if you've ever been on a diet that required you to count every single calorie you put in your mouth, the chances are you were doomed to failure from the start. Sure the quantity you consume is important but cutting calories isn't always the answer and you don't have to count every single one. In fact you may not have to change the quantity at all. In my experience I've come across just as many people not eating enough as eating too much.

Frankly, the prospect of having to add up and keep score of every calorie that I consume on a daily basis for the rest of my life bores me to tears. So I don't want you to do it either. Remember how I said that it's very difficult to over-eat protein or fat but it's very easy to over-eat carbohydrates (think back to the bath). If your diet is lower in processed foods and simple carbs, the chances are you will find it much harder to over-eat anyway.

There is, however, the issue of not eating enough and that's pretty important. Remember you need fuel and the more you move the more fuel you need. This whole process is called your metabolism – the rate at which your body burns energy. If you feed your body with only a small amount of food each day, you may not be giving your body enough for even its most basic functions. Over time your body will have to break down some of your muscle tissue to make up the shortfall, which can damage your metabolism and affect the rate at which you store fat. This is your body's survival mechanism to keep you alive in times of famine.

One of the aims of this book is to help you make some changes to the way you eat, what you eat and the food habits you have formed over time. If you are already getting your diet half-right, the healthy eating plan that follows will help to eliminate those bad habits altogether. If you think you need a lot more help with your diet, the plan will act as a starting point. The right combination of foods required for optimal health can differ from person to person and you may need to experiment a little to get things right for you but, ultimately, embracing a healthier way of eating is a great place to start.

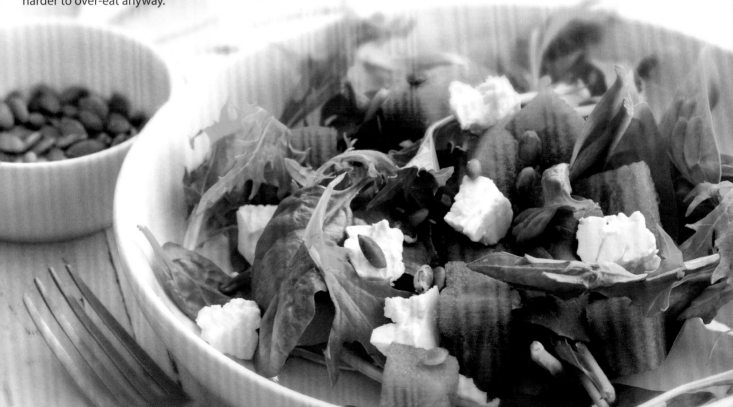

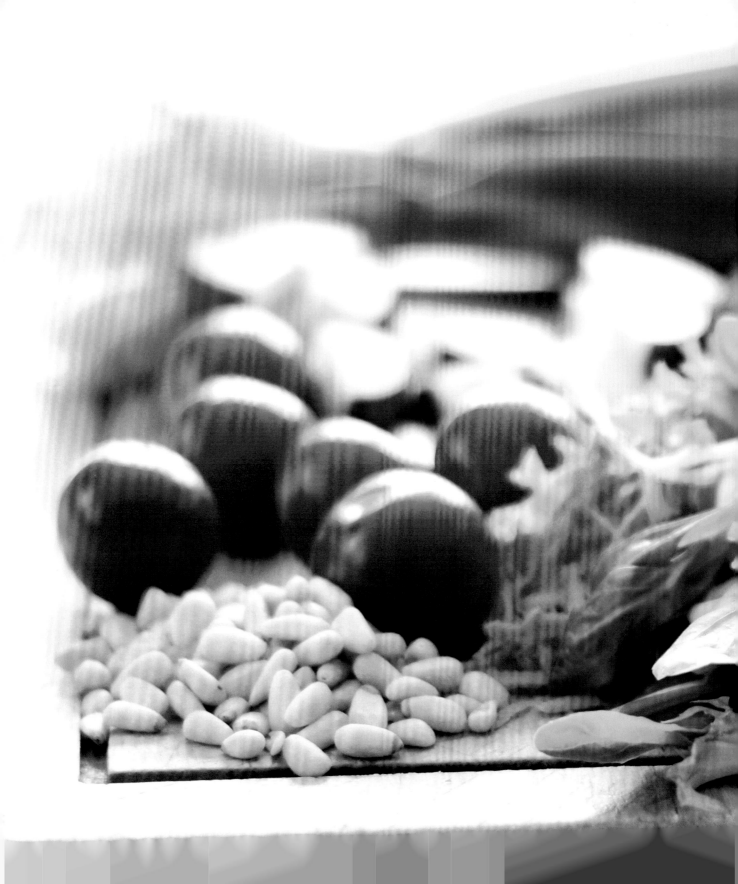

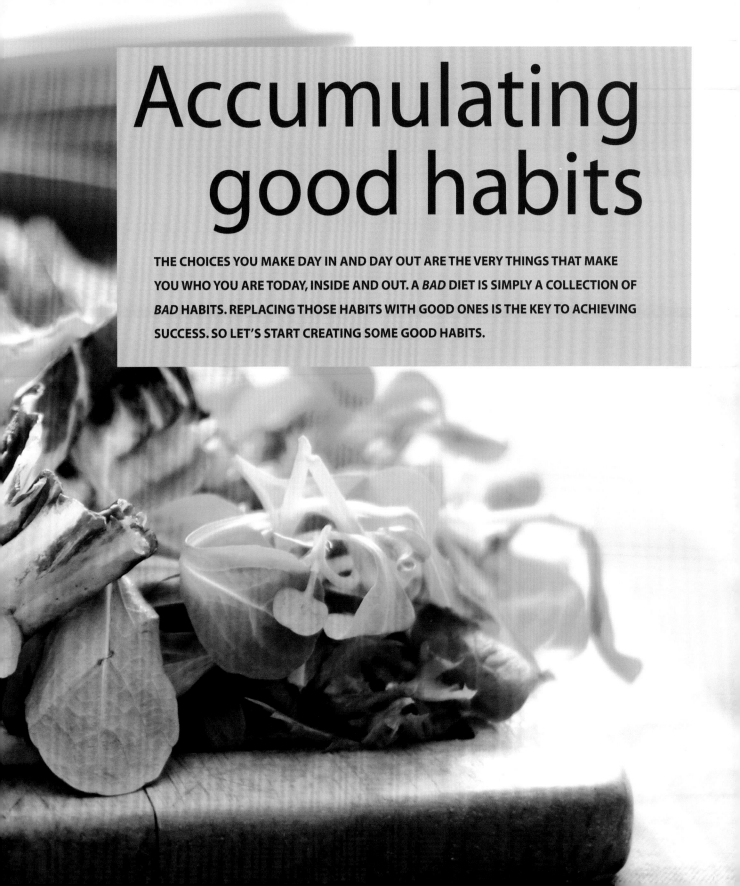

Accumulating good habits

THE CHOICES YOU MAKE DAY IN AND DAY OUT ARE THE VERY THINGS THAT MAKE YOU WHO YOU ARE TODAY, INSIDE AND OUT. A *BAD* DIET IS SIMPLY A COLLECTION OF *BAD* HABITS. REPLACING THOSE HABITS WITH GOOD ONES IS THE KEY TO ACHIEVING SUCCESS. SO LET'S START CREATING SOME GOOD HABITS.

The Accumulator™ 30-day healthy habits plan

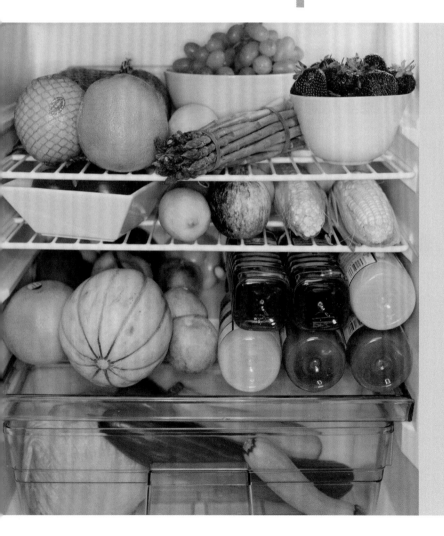

NOT ONLY DOES THIS BOOK COME WITH A WORKOUT PLAN, THE ACCUMULATOR™ WILL ALSO HELP YOU TO CREATE GOOD DIETARY PRACTICES AND ELIMINATE BAD ONES. IN ORDER TO MAKE ANY CHANGE TO YOUR BEHAVIOUR AND TURN IT INTO A HABIT YOU NEED TO DO IT OVER AND OVER AGAIN. THERE'S A COMMON BELIEF, MADE POPULAR BY MAXWELL MALTZ WHO WROTE ABOUT IT IN HIS 1960 BOOK ON SELF-IMAGE *PSYCHO-CYBERNETICS*, THAT CREATING A NEW HABIT TAKES ONLY 21 DAYS.

MY EXPERIENCE IS THAT IT CAN VARY WILDLY DEPENDING ON THE PERSON AND CIRCUMSTANCES BUT IN GENERAL IF YOU CAN DO SOMETHING EVERY DAY FOR A MONTH THERE'S A PRETTY GOOD CHANCE YOU'LL KEEP DOING IT.

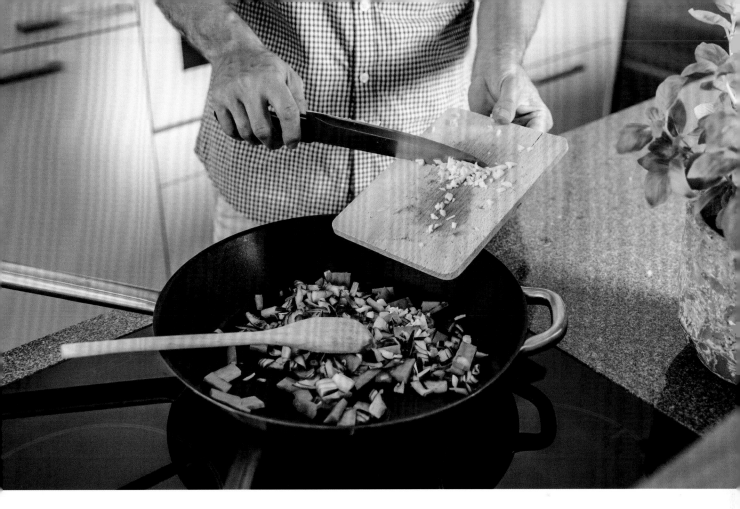

With this in mind, I've created a 30-day plan that enables you to incorporate good eating habits into your routine. A lot of these are nothing more than common sense. Over the course of 30 days I will ask you to make one change in relation to your diet each day. So on Day 1 you only need to change one thing. On Day 2 I will set you a new task and then we'll to go back over the change you made on the previous day just to make sure that's still in place. This continues over the 30 days. By Day 30 you will have been doing some of these things for several weeks and they should already be turning into habits. In fact, you will have been doing them for so long that you may not even realise you're still doing some of them at all.

Once the 30 days are over, simply keep all of your new habits in place for ever and you will, without doubt, have made a massive impact on the way you eat and the way you

LEFT AND ABOVE Slowly start incorporating healthy habits into your routine.

look in the mirror. Be aware though that you may need to make further modifications to the diet you eat in order to achieve your own specific weight-loss goals. There may also be some advice here that will not be appropriate for you due to existing restrictions or special considerations within your diet. As with exercise, the way you eat will be unique to you and some of the habits I suggest here may not be ideal for you. If you are in any doubt, it is best to check with a doctor or nutritionist before you begin.

Before you begin though, I'd like you to take a snapshot of the way you eat right now. In fact, I want you to take several snapshots. Continue eating as you already do for the next two days, taking a photo of each item before you eat it.

DAY 1

Make your kitchen healthy

THIS IS ONE OF THE BEST HABITS YOU CAN INCLUDE IN YOUR MONTHLY ROUTINE TO PREVENT YOU FROM SUCCUMBING TO TEMPTATION, WHICH IS WHY WE'RE DOING IT ON DAY 1. HAVE YOU EVER FELT THE NEED FOR SOMETHING TO EAT BUT YOU'RE NOT REALLY THAT HUNGRY? YOU KNOW, THAT MOMENT WHEN YOU'RE PERHAPS A LITTLE BORED, NEED A DISTRACTION OR YOU MAY BE FEELING A LITTLE LOW. YOU HEAD TO THE FRIDGE, OPEN IT AND SEE IF THERE'S ANYTHING YOU FANCY. YOU MAY EVEN GO BACK TWO OR THREE TIMES MORE JUST IN CASE THERE'S A TASTY TREAT LURKING IN THE CORNER.

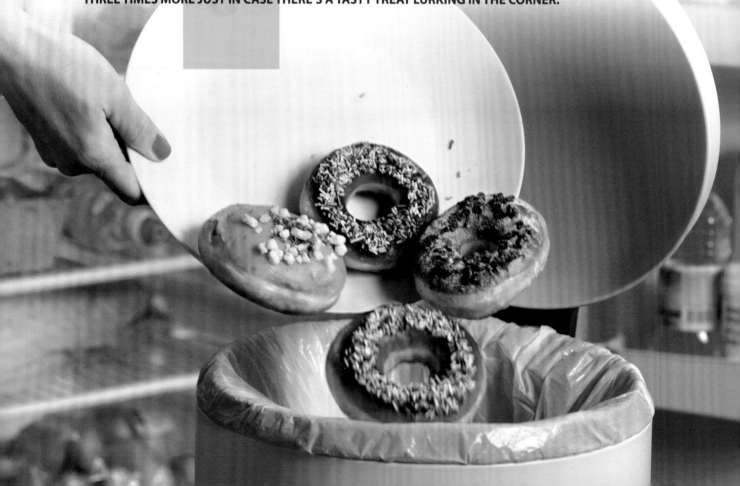

RESIST THE URGE TO SNACK

We all have moments in our day that spark the desire for food that we simply don't need. Sitting in front of the TV for instance, or perhaps for you it's that hour after the kids come home from school. If there's something unhealthy in the kitchen during these times we will usually go for the worst thing we can find. Even if it's the last, slightly soft cookie lingering at the bottom of the jar, that will do just fine.

Trying to override whatever triggers that urge to snack is sometimes the hardest habit to break. Personally, I get the temptation to raid the fridge when I'm writing, but I'm happy to say I don't give in.

remove
temptation!

DITCH THE JUNK The easiest way to remove temptation and make sure you still get something to eat is to keep your kitchen healthy. This may be tough, but take a deep breath and get it done. Grab a bin liner and go through your fridge, freezer, larder, kitchen cupboards – anywhere you keep food.

Now throw away anything you feel will become an unhealthy temptation during those moments of weakness ... and I mean anything. Remember, don't just tip it in the bin – make sure you recycle everything. And by that I don't mean eating all the unhealthy food in your house before starting this plan – all you'd be doing is putting it off and adding to the problems that led you to buying this book in the first place – throw it out or give it away, just get it out of your house. If there's no junk food in the kitchen, you can't eat any.

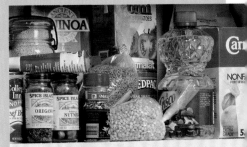
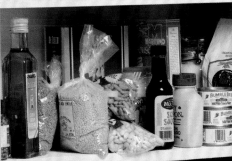
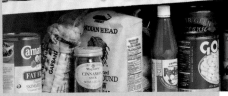

eat
enough

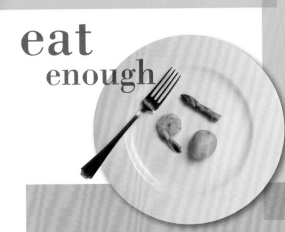

DON'T STARVE YOURSELF Of course it may not just be a habit or our mood that triggers the need for a sweet treat. For many, wanting a sugary snack can be a result of not having eaten enough.

Remember the bath metaphor we covered in the last chapter? When your body's energy stores are low you will crave something sweet so you get the fuel you need as soon as possible. So you could be a habit snacker, an undernourished snacker or, even worse, both.

override
triggers that
urge you to snack!

DAY 2

Keep a shopping list

NOW YOU HAVE NOTHING IN YOUR CUPBOARDS BECAUSE SOME IDIOT IN A BOOK TOLD YOU TO THROW IT ALL AWAY. SO IT'S TIME TO GO SHOPPING. NOW, BEFORE YOU JUMP IN THE CAR AND HEAD AIMLESSLY FOR THE SHOPS, YOU NEED TO HAVE A PLAN. MAKING A SHOPPING LIST IS ONE OF THE BEST THINGS YOU CAN DO TO KEEP YOU FROM REPLACING ALL THE FOODSTUFFS YOU THREW OUT YESTERDAY WITH MORE UNHEALTHY ONES. OFTEN PEOPLE BUY MANY OF THE SAME THINGS WEEK AFTER WEEK AND SOME OF THE UNHEALTHY OPTIONS IN YOUR BASKET MAY JUST BE HABIT BUYS.

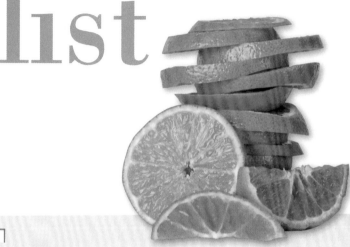

BRING ON THE NUTRIENTS Now is your chance to think about replacing those unhealthy foods with good ones. Go back to the previous chapter to help you decide what you're going to put on your list. Think about the meals you're going to make and what ingredients you'll need to make them. Replace the treats you have in those moments of weakness with nutritious alternatives.

Fill your shopping list with food and not products made with food. Once you have your list then keep that list as a basis for your next grocery shop. Pin it to your fridge or somewhere you can get to it every day. I have a blackboard in my kitchen for new items and split my main list into different meals or different types of food. I make a carbohydrate list, a protein list, a list for fruit and a snack list and so on.

A quick recap

☑ *Keep your kitchen healthy.*

Before we've finished with Day 2, don't forget to make sure your kitchen is still healthy. If you live alone, this won't be a problem, but if you're not the only one who brings food through the door then some unhealthy things may have made their way into your fridge, which could lead to trouble when you get a craving.

Now would be a good time to sit down with your family or the other people that share your home and ask for their help. Tell them what you're doing and why, and request that if they buy anything they store it somewhere where you can't get at it. Better still, bring them all along for the ride. If your entire household supports each other with this month of change, your success rate will soar.

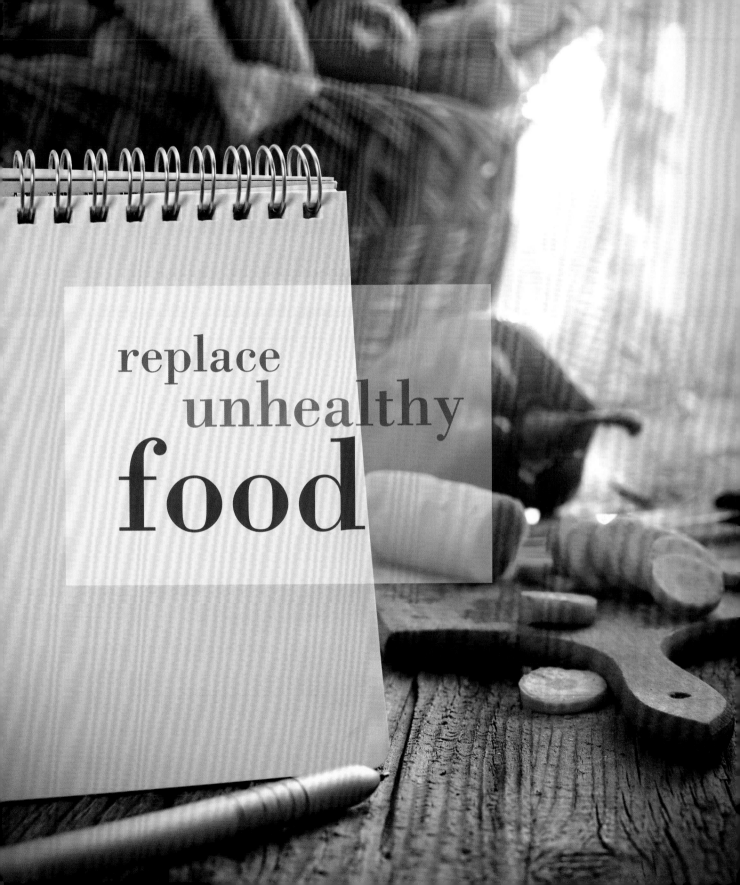

replace
unhealthy
food

DAY 3

Plan your meals

A LACK OF PLANNING MAY RESULT IN YOU MAKING A BAD DECISION. THIS IS PARTICULARLY TRUE WHEN IT COMES TO FOOD. YOU WILL HAVE ALREADY STARTED TO THINK ABOUT THIS YESTERDAY, BUT TODAY I'D LIKE YOU TO DO A LITTLE RESEARCH. I COULD EASILY LIST LOTS OF HEALTHY RECIPES AT THIS POINT BUT, TO BE PERFECTLY HONEST, THAT'S NOT WHAT THIS BOOK IS ABOUT AND I'M NO GOURMET CHEF. MAKING YOUR OWN INFORMED CHOICES ABOUT YOUR MEALS IS A MUCH MORE EFFECTIVE WAY TO ENSURE YOU STAY ON TRACK ANYWAY. HOWEVER, DON'T FORGET THAT THIS BOOK COMES WITH LOTS OF EXTRA RESOURCES AT WWW.THEACCUMULATOR.NET AND THERE ARE PLENTY OF HEALTHY MEAL IDEAS THERE TO GET YOU STARTED.

KEEP IT SIMPLE As long as you stick to my laws of food you'll have plenty of scope to be creative. If you're no genius in the kitchen (like me), keep it simple, but do experiment. I don't expect you to be eating the best diet for you within a week or even a month, but at least you are making some positive changes.

A quick recap

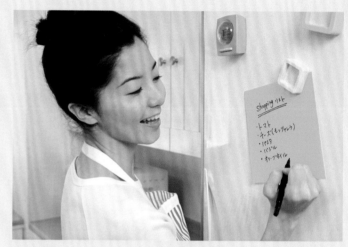

☑ Keep a shopping list

Where is it? You pinned it on your fridge or kept it somewhere you could get at it, didn't you? Take a quick look and make sure there's nothing missing for your next shopping trip. The chances are that while you're experimenting you may find yourself food shopping more than once per week, but once this period of change settles into a routine you should be going once each week for most items and perhaps a little more frequently for fresh food.

☑ Keep your kitchen healthy

Is there still something unhealthy in your kitchen that's becoming a draw in those moments of weakness? Three days in and your taste buds may have discovered something new but just as unhealthy as the food you threw out. Remember to keep your kitchen healthy.

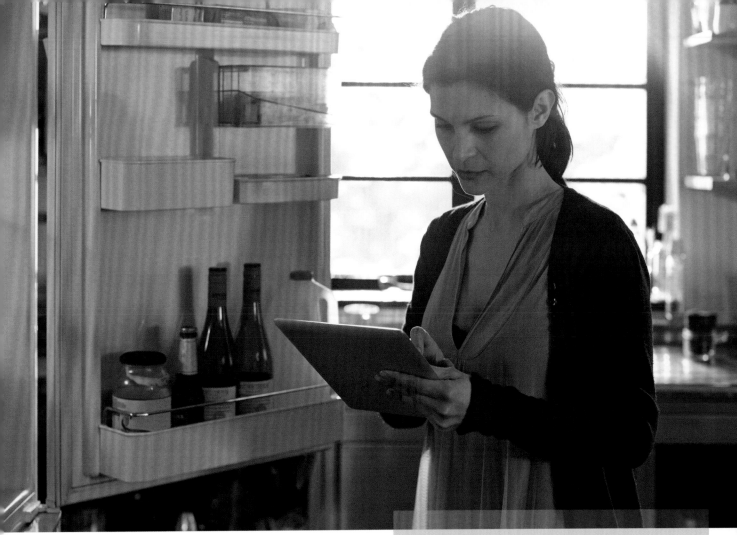

shop frequently
for fresh
food

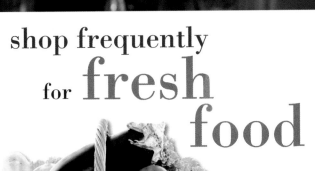

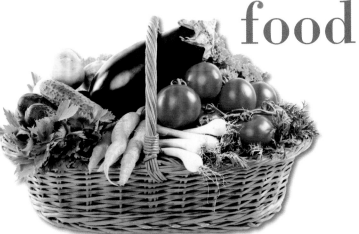

MAKE SURE YOU HAVE ALL THAT YOU NEED Think baby steps and not giant leaps to success. Keep meal planning on your radar and you'll accumulate a library of tasty, healthy meal options in no time.

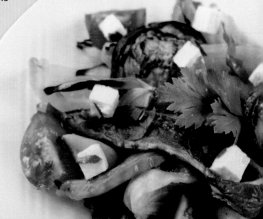

DAY 4

Never go hungry

LET'S GO BACK TO THE BATH METAPHOR AND ADD ONE MORE SCENARIO TO THE LIST. THIS TIME YOU'RE NOT FILLING YOUR BATH WITH ONLY CARBOHYDRATES BUT WITH ALL THE FOOD YOU EAT IN A DAY. THE PLUG IS NOW HALF IN AND HALF OUT SO THE WATER IS FILLING UP BUT IT'S ALWAYS EMPTYING A LITTLE AT THE SAME TIME. IF YOU MANAGE TO GET THE FLOW OF WATER JUST RIGHT, YOU'LL ATTAIN EQUILIBRIUM. THE BATH WATER WILL ALWAYS BE AT THE SAME LEVEL – IT WILL NEVER BE EMPTY AND IT WILL NEVER BE FULL. THEN AT THE END OF THE DAY YOU CAN TURN OFF THE TAPS AND LET THE WATER DRAIN AWAY. THIS IS THE BEST WAY TO THINK ABOUT YOUR FOOD INTAKE EACH DAY. YOU SHOULD NEVER GO HUNGRY BUT AT THE SAME TIME YOU SHOULD NEVER BE IN THAT UNCOMFORTABLE POSITION WHEN YOU FEEL SO STUFFED THAT YOU HAVE TO UNDO YOUR TROUSERS SO YOU CAN BREATHE.

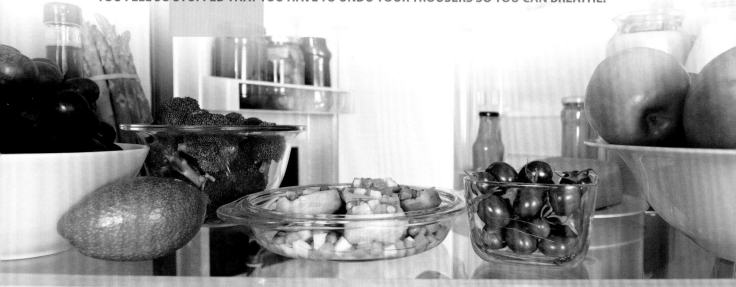

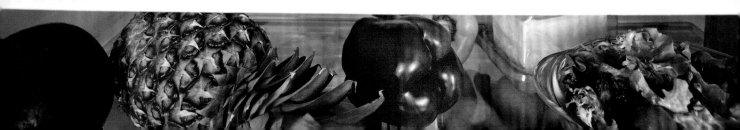

are you really hungry?

Many people don't eat a thing until lunchtime and then save themselves for a huge meal eaten only a few hours before going to bed. This can have a damaging effect on your metabolism and cause you to make some bad food choices.

Eating regularly works well in two ways: first, it helps to regulate some of the hormones in your body that are triggered when you eat something, so they can now work at the same level all day rather than having to work extra hard for one part of the day and not at all for the rest; second, this habit also works to ward off temptation.

Remember Day 1? Feeling hungry is your body's way of telling you that you need something to fill that void, and that's when you're more likely to make bad decisions if there are no healthy options available (remember to keep your kitchen healthy). Bear in mind, though, that this is not a green light to eat more, just to keep hunger at bay.

FAST OVERNIGHT It's also important to make sure your bath is empty for a while too. Overnight fasting for around 12 hours will allow your digestive system to recover and re-set. If you usually have breakfast at 7 a.m., make sure you close down the kitchen after 7 p.m. the previous evening. It's important, too, not to confuse hunger with something else, such as thirst, boredom or just a food craving. If you usually snack in front of the TV in the evening and start feeling hungry at this time, are you really hungry? Try drinking a glass of water first just to be sure the feeling is not just thirst.

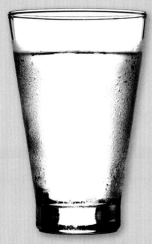

A quick recap

☑ Plan your meals

Make sure you end each day by planning for the next one. If you have to eat lunch away from home, do you know what you're going to have? Have you prepared something to take with you? A packed lunch prepared the day before ensures you're not going to make a bad choice when it comes to lunch the following day. Do you have anything frozen that needs defrosting before you can eat it? If so, get it out and ready before you leave for work. Be constantly looking out for healthy meal ideas. The more you think about healthy eating the more you will see it around you and the more likely you are to do it.

☑ Keep a shopping list

If you've run out of anything, put it on the list or go out and get it. Have you seen a new recipe you'd like to try? Make sure anything you need goes on the list.

☑ Keep your kitchen healthy

If you've been a sugar junkie up until now, you may find you will be looking out for something sweet to eat today. Remember, if there's processed food lurking your kitchen, remove it from the house.

keep hunger away!

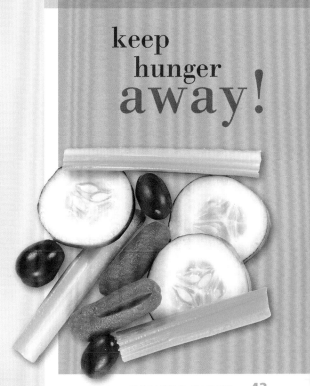

DAY 5 Break the fast

BY NOW YOU SHOULD BE AT A POINT WHERE YOU HAVE STOPPED COMFORT EATING IN FRONT OF THE TV OR TUCKING INTO A LATE-NIGHT MEAL. WHEN YOU WAKE UP IN THE MORNING, THEREFORE, YOU WILL HAVE BEEN WITHOUT FOOD FOR AROUND 12 HOURS. YOU NEED SOMETHING TO BREAK THE FAST: BREAKFAST. IT DOES WHAT IT SAYS IT DOES. SKIPPING BREAKFAST IS A SURE-FIRE ROUTE TO GAINING WEIGHT, AS IS SKIPPING ANY MEAL. IF YOU'RE NOT USED TO EATING SOMETHING FIRST THING YOU PROBABLY DON'T WAKE UP HUNGRY, RIGHT? THAT'S BECAUSE YOUR BODY IS USED TO FENDING FOR ITSELF AND NOT BECAUSE YOU DON'T NEED ANYTHING TO EAT.

think simple, think food!

don't skip
meals

WAKE UP YOUR METABOLISM

You body requires something for your metabolism to do, something to wake up your hormones and start regulating your system for another day. You need water in your bath. Skipping breakfast will also leave you wide open to temptation later in the morning as your body starts to crave the easiest source of energy it can find.

is your list looking different?

BRING ON BREAKFAST
If you don't normally eat breakfast, start with something small and simple and slowly build it up as your metabolism gets used to having something to do each morning. I don't expect you to have a big bowl of porridge or smoked salmon on your first day, as you may feel ill if you do. Ideally, as with any meal, breakfast should be a mixture of macronutrients and follow all the laws of food. Unfortunately, for many people, this meal is a processed-food party consisting of sugar-laden cereals and juice, refined treated dairy products, preservative-filled bread and caffeine. Think simple, think food and you can't go very wrong. Above all, make time for breakfast.

A quick recap

☑ **Never go hungry**

If you're out for the day, have you made any provision to avoid hunger? Are you taking enough food with you? Do you have something unprocessed and non-perishable in the car in case you end up stuck in traffic?

☑ **Plan your meals**

You should have already done this last night, and you'll need to make sure you do it tonight for tomorrow's meals. Remember, fail to plan and you can plan to fail. Make sure you have lunch sorted, especially if you'll be away from home. Do you know what you're eating tomorrow evening? Do you have everything in your fridge to make it?

☑ **Keep a shopping list**

See how it flows so nicely? If you're working down this list (as I hope you are) you should already have in your mind some things that need to go on your shopping list. In fact, the list you made on Day 1 may be looking a little different from the one you have now.

☑ **Keep your kitchen healthy**

Not only should there be no junk in your kitchen but your kitchen should be clean. There's nothing worse than going into the kitchen in the morning to find there are dishes to be done or things to tidy up. That all takes time to sort out, and time can be at a premium first thing in the morning and you need enough of it to eat a healthy breakfast and make sure your lunch is sorted. So, spend five minutes at the end of every evening making your kitchen morning-ready.

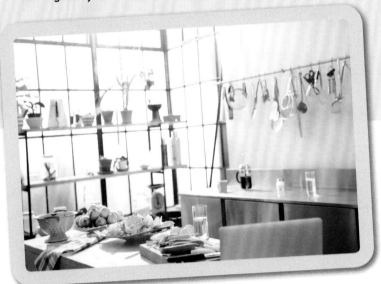

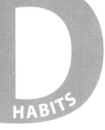

Take the measure of your meals

REMEMBER, IT'S QUALITY AND NOT QUANTITY THAT'S IMPORTANT WHEN IT COMES TO YOUR DAILY DIET. NOT ONLY DOES THAT INCLUDE MAKING SURE THE FOOD ON YOUR PLATE IS OF THE BEST STANDARD (SEE THE LAWS OF FOOD), IT ALSO MEANS THAT YOU HAVE THE RIGHT COMBINATION IN THE RIGHT QUANTITIES. TODAY, FOCUS ON THE TYPES OF FOOD YOU HAVE ON YOUR PLATE. TAKE A LOOK AT WHAT YOU'RE EATING; DO YOU KNOW HOW MUCH OF EACH OF THE MACRONUTRIENTS ESSENTIAL FOR A HEALTHY DIET ARE ON YOUR PLATE?

get the
balance
right

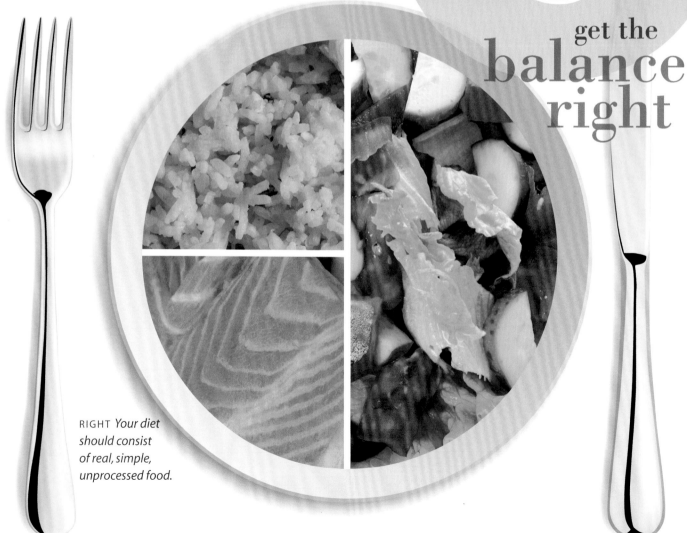

RIGHT *Your diet should consist of real, simple, unprocessed food.*

the macronutrients

PROTEIN: First off, about a quarter of your plate should consist of lean protein. Take a look at the previous chapter (see page 30) and see if there's anything on your plate that fits the bill.

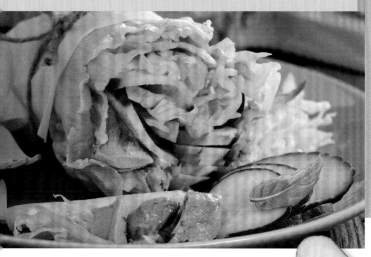

CARBOHYDRATE: Is there any complex carbohydrate on your plate (the low-GI foods that keep your energy levels up for longer)? This should not take up more than a quarter of your plate.

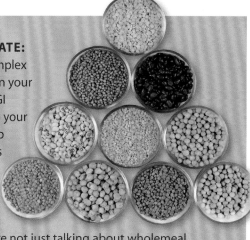

Remember we're not just talking about wholemeal bread, pasta and rice here – squashes, sweet potatoes, beans, lentils and quinoa should be higher on your list of everyday carbs. Lentils and quinoa have the added benefit of containing protein as well as carbohydrate.

VEGETABLES: Fill the rest of your plate with fresh veggies, salad or root vegetables (but not potato).

FATS: A small amount of olive oil, coconut oil, oily fish, avocados, nuts, seeds or dairy products (preferably organic) should appear somewhere on the plate. These foods have the added benefit of making you feel fuller for longer as well as making food more palatable and keeping your body functioning properly.

A quick recap

☑ Break the fast

If you're not used to eating anything in the morning this is going to take time to get used to. If you're a habitual sugar-consumer at breakfast, start to experiment with different things so you have a more balanced plate. Think simple, real, healthy, unprocessed food. Most important of all, make time for breakfast.

☑ Never go hungry

If you're finding yourself getting hungry by lunchtime or in need of something in the afternoon, make sure there's a healthy snack available to keep you going. If you're used to only three or even only two meals per day, you might feel like you don't need anything in between. However, if you've made some big changes to your diet and started exercising more, you may find in the coming weeks that you feel hungry more often.

☑ Plan your meals

Are you set for tomorrow? Do you know what you're going to eat?

☑ Keep a shopping list

It should be right there on your fridge. I take a photo of mine with my phone before heading out to the shops.

☑ Keep your kitchen healthy

You shouldn't need to do an actual check at all by now but, just in case, have a quick look.

It's treat day

YES, YOU DID READ THAT CORRECTLY. THIS DOESN'T MEAN THAT YOU CAN FORGET DAYS 1–6 AND TOTALLY LET YOUR HAIR DOWN; THIS IS ONE TREAT AND NOT A JUNK-FOOD BINGE. FOR ANY EATING PLAN TO BE A PRACTICAL AND VIABLE OPTION IN THE LONG TERM YOU HAVE TO FACTOR IN A LITTLE OF SOMETHING YOU FANCY NOW AND AGAIN. THE UNHEALTHY FOODS THAT YOU REALLY LOVE WILL BE IMPOSSIBLE TO RESIST IF YOU TRY TO REMOVE THEM FROM YOUR LIFE COMPLETELY, AND YOU MAY END UP OVER-EATING THEM TO COMPENSATE AND FEEING LIKE A FAILURE.

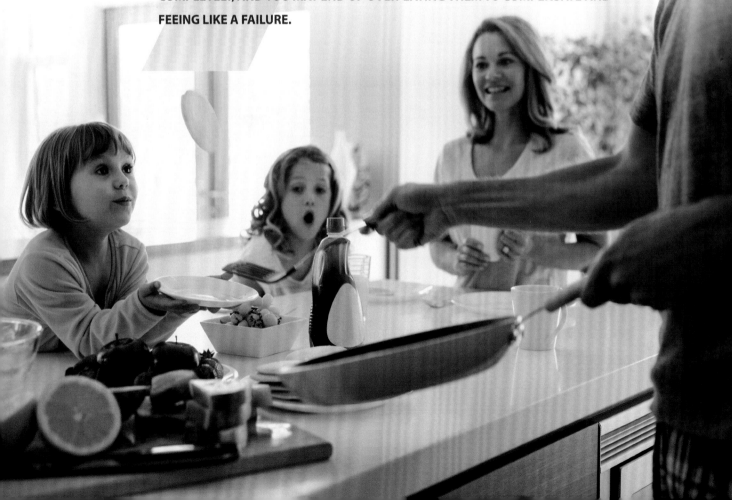

don't forget
to eat!

TIME FOR A TREAT Don't totally eliminate treats from your diet, just enjoy them occasionally on an allocated treat day. Mine is always a Saturday and my treat is either my evening meal or something sweet afterwards. Sometimes, though, I may be invited out or feel the need to have my treat day at another time during the week, in which case I simply make a trade and stick to my normal eating habits that weekend. So allow yourself one treat each week on your shopping list or indulge if a little if you go out for a meal.

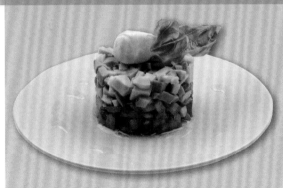

DON'T SABOTAGE YOURSELF
Don't use your treat day as an excuse to overeat. If you are planning an indulgent evening meal, don't be tempted to skip food earlier in the day as this can lead to overeating all the wrong things.

A quick recap

☑ **Take the measure of your meals**
If you're having a meal as a treat today you can ignore this rule, but for the rest of the day it still applies. Keep an eye on your checklist to be sure you have all these elements on your plate: protein – keep it lean and making up around a quarter of your plate; carbohydrate – complex and not simple, remember some colour too; fats – does anything on your plate contain fat? If not, add a little in.

☑ **Break the fast**
Your treat should not be staying in bed until lunchtime and skipping breakfast. Remember, you need to break the fast. In fact, breakfast can even be your treat meal. Pancakes anyone?

☑ **Never go hungry**
If you're like most people, your habits change over the weekend and healthy eating can easily be forgotten. If you started Day 1 on Monday then today is Sunday and you might find many of your good intentions go out of the window. You may also be so busy or having such a good time that you forget to eat. However ...

☑ **Plan your meals**
... if you planned yesterday, this won't be a problem. You still need to be prepared for tomorrow though, especially if you're returning to your weekday routine.

☑ **Keep a shopping list**
Check your cupboards and make sure nothing is missing.

☑ **Keep your kitchen healthy**
While you are checking your cupboards for ingredients, make sure there are no unhealthy treats left to tempt you tomorrow.

don't
forget!
Remove the unhealthy treats for tomorrow!

DAY 8

Go green

VEGGIES SHOULD ALREADY BE A BIG PART OF YOUR DIET BUT TODAY YOU ARE GOING TO UP YOUR QUOTA OF FIBRE, VITAMINS AND MINERALS BY ADDING SOMETHING GREEN TO AT LEAST TWO OF YOUR MEALS OR SNACKS. GREAT GREEN FOODS INCLUDE: AVOCADOS, SPINACH, KALE, SPROUTS, CUCUMBERS, CELERY, PEAS, APPLES, KIWIS, MELONS, GREEN TEA, GREEN (BELL) PEPPERS, GREEN CHILLIES, ASPARAGUS, PISTACHIO NUTS, MINT.

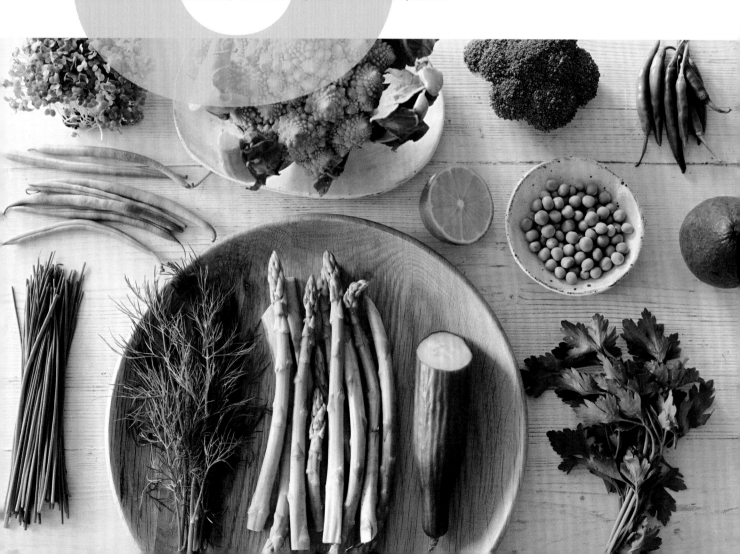

keep everything
junk free

try green tea
with a dash
of lemon

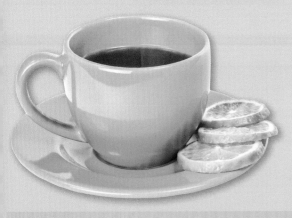

EAT GREEN Green, leafy vegetables contain a chemical called chlorophyll, which makes them green. Chlorophyll is great at keeping our red blood cells healthy and can protect against many diseases including some cancers. You'll also find plenty of vitamins, folic acid, iron, calcium, protein and antioxidants in natural green foods.

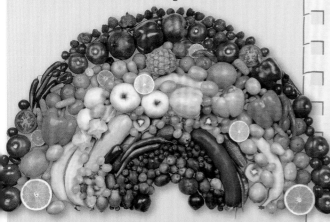

add.
spices
to make your
food tasty

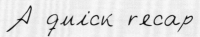

A quick recap

☑ **Take the measure of your meals**

Remember this one? Keep a check on what's on your plate and make sure there's a little bit of everything. Protein, carbohydrate and a little fat.

☑ **Break the fast**

As we head into week 2 you should already be waking up looking forward to breakfast. You will probably have expanded your repertoire and begun experimenting. So many people stick to the same thing for breakfast, meaning it can easily become the most boring meal of the day. So, if you haven't already done so, try spicing things up a little and plan three different breakfasts for the week.

☑ **Never go hungry**

If today is a busy one, be prepared in case you get hungry. Remember not to confuse hunger with something else, such as thirst.

☑ **Plan your meals**

Start thinking about something different for breakfast (see above). Add green foods to your meals and spice up snacks.

☑ **Keep a shopping list**

Remember that I suggested you split up your list into smaller sub-lists for each meal or type of food? Try to add something new to each sub-list today, or pick up something new at the supermarket.

☑ **Keep your kitchen healthy**

Keep everything junk free.

DAY 9

Go nuts

EATING NUTS (AND SEEDS) IS A GREAT WAY TO GET A HIT OF PROTEIN AT SNACK TIME AND YOU DON'T NEED MANY TO FILL YOU UP. MOREOVER, THEY ARE PACKED WITH MANY ESSENTIAL NUTRIENTS. AS WITH ANY FOOD, THE NUTS YOU CHOOSE NEED TO BE NATURAL, BY WHICH I MEAN NOT ROASTED IN OIL OR SMOTHERED IN SALT OR OTHER FLAVOURS. EAT THEM RAW INSTEAD AND GO FOR ALMONDS, CASHEW NUTS, PISTACHIOS, WALNUTS AND A FEW BRAZIL NUTS (THESE ARE FULL OF SELENIUM, WHICH CAN BE GOOD FOR PROSTATE HEALTH). TRY TO KEEP MACADAMIAS, PECAN NUTS AND PEANUTS TO A MINIMUM (PEANUTS AREN'T ACTUALLY NUTS ANYWAY, THEY ARE LEGUMES SINCE THEY GROW UNDERGROUND).

MIX IT UP! You can mix your nuts up with pumpkin seeds and sunflower seeds. I'm lucky enough to have a good market nearby where I can pick and mix my own bag of nuts and seeds. Most supermarkets sell individual bags of nuts that you can mix together, which is usually a better option than the pre-mixed selections that may contain lots of high-sugar dried fruit. Antioxidant-rich dried goji berries (right) also make a great addition to your mix. NB: some people do have intolerances or even allergies to some nuts. Obviously if this applies to you then steer well clear of them.

keep macadamias, pecan nuts & peanuts to a minimum

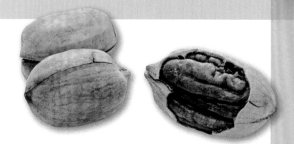

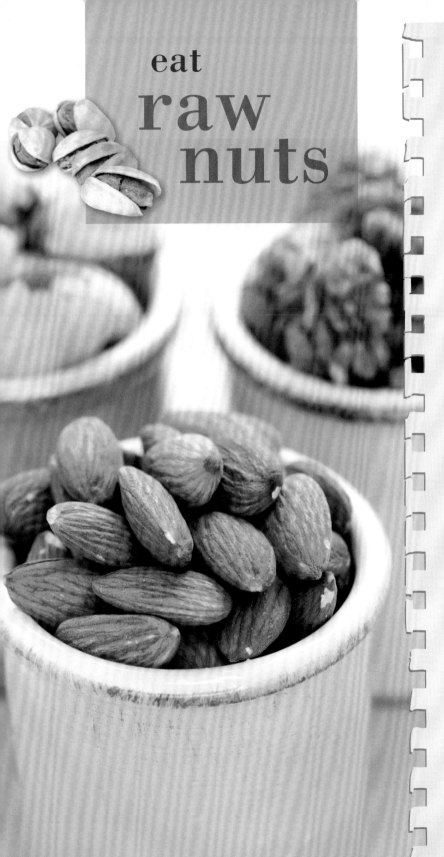

eat
raw
nuts

A quick recap

☑ **Go green**

Don't forget to put something green on your plate – it could be some pistachio nuts since we are discussing nuts today.

☑ **Take the measure of your meals and break the fast**

☑ **Never go hungry**

Pack a handful of nuts into a sealed bag or pot and take them with you when you go out.

☑ **Plan your meals**

Why not look up a new recipe for tomorrow that contains nuts?

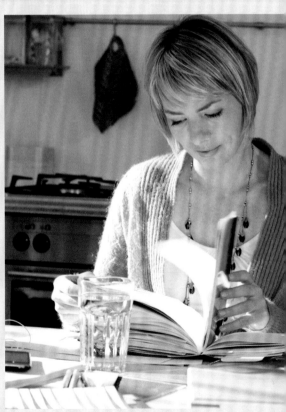

☑ **Keep a shopping list**

Now you can add nuts, seeds and even some goji berries to your list.

☑ **Keep your kitchen healthy**

DAY 10

Practise smart eating

THIS ISN'T NECESSARILY A PRACTICE YOU WILL NEED TO DO TODAY, BUT IT IS SOMETHING THAT'S IMPORTANT TO BE AWARE OF AND CERTAINLY A HABIT YOU WILL NEED IN YOUR LIFE. WHEN YOU GO OUT FOR A MEAL, REMEMBER THAT YOU DON'T NEED TO ABANDON ALL THE GOOD HABITS YOU'RE NOW STARTING TO ESTABLISH.

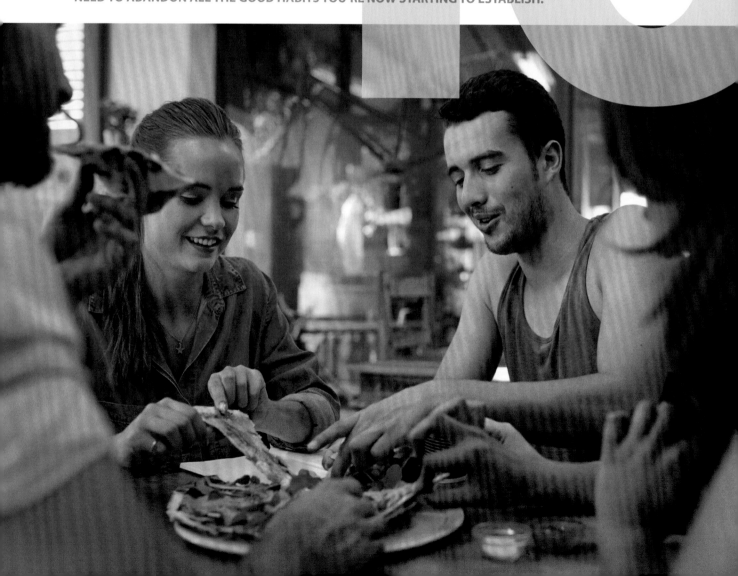

tips to ensure you don't fall off the wagon when you eat out

1

ORDER AN APPETISER AND SALAD as your main meal or share an appetiser and eat a small main course.

2

IF YOU ORDER SALAD, ask for the dressing to be served separately so you can control the quantity you apply.

3

GRILLED, BAKED OR ROASTED poultry breast, fish and shellfish are good choices as they are packed with protein, vitamins and minerals and the latter contain beneficial fats.

4

IF YOU HAVE A SAUCE, opt for simple tomato based ones rather than something more processed.

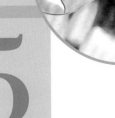

5

REMEMBER DESSERT COULD BE A TREAT or you could opt for a fruit salad or sorbet.

A quick recap

☑ **Go nuts**
Nuts can be great as part of a meal and not just as a snack. I always sprinkle some in a salad, add them to chilli con carne and I use ground almonds as a batter for fish.

☑ **Go green**
Be creative here, too. How about some grated apple in porridge? Or chop up some celery to add some crunch to a stir-fry, or stuff a pepper.

☑ **Take the measure of your meals**
Make sure you're still getting all the protein, carbs and fat that you need. It's very easy to slip back into your old ways and eat a plate of carbohydrates without even realising.

☑ **Break the fast**
If you're in a rush something is always better than nothing, even if you grab a piece of fruit before heading out of the door. If you find you're pressed for time at breakfast on a regular basis, maybe think about being prepared. Have something made and ready the night before that you can take with you if you need it.

☑ **Never go hungry**
With the exercise you're doing, you may find your metabolism has been given a boost and your body will need extra food to keep hunger at bay, but if you're eating more protein than you were when you started the plan, you should feel satiated for longer.

☑ **Plan your meals**

☑ **Keep a shopping list**
Your shopping list should be very different now and you may even want to think about looking beyond the supermarket for your groceries. Is there a farm shop or farmer's market near you? A local butcher or fishmonger could be a better option than a supermarket, too, as the food may be fresher and you can choose the best cuts.

☑ **Keep your kitchen healthy**
If you have kids (or a significant other), they may not be playing by the same rules as you. If they bring something unhealthy into the house, try to re-educate them or, at the very least, make sure they keep it out of your reach. If you were a sugar addict, you may even find that your taste buds are starting to change.

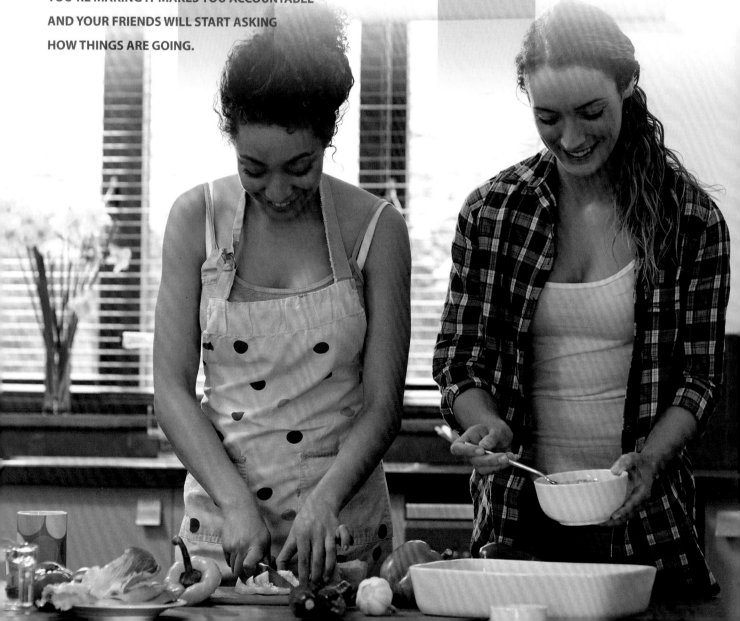

DAY 1

HABITS

Show your support

THE BEST WAY TO ENSURE YOU STICK TO THE NEW HABITS YOU'RE CREATING IS TO TALK ABOUT THEM. AS SOON AS YOU TELL YOUR FAMILY AND FRIENDS ABOUT THE CHANGES YOU'RE MAKING IT MAKES YOU ACCOUNTABLE AND YOUR FRIENDS WILL START ASKING HOW THINGS ARE GOING.

A quick recap

☑ Practise smart eating

If you plan to eat out today, make sure you plan. No matter where you go, you will still be able to make your meal out a healthy one that won't break any of the other good habits you're building on this month. Make sure you go over the tips from Day 10 and you can't go too wrong. As this plan progresses you will discover that the way you think about food will naturally change and you'll automatically make better choices when it comes to eating out.

☑ Go nuts

Eat some as a snack or incorporate nuts and seeds into one of your main meals. I always have a small bag in my car in case I'm caught out and become hungry. There's nothing worse than sitting in traffic for hours with your stomach rumbling.

☑ Go green

Is there something green on your plate? How about adding in something green you haven't already tried? It's true that some foods are an acquired taste and this may apply to you. I used to have a real problem with spinach. Even as a kid, Popeye could not convince me to eat the stuff. Now I grow my own and eat it almost every day.

☑ Take the measure of your meals

When preparing a meal, ask yourself if you've included all the components. Pretty soon you'll do this automatically.

☑ Break the fast

If you know you are going to be in a rush the following morning, how about preparing something the night before? Remember the 12-hour fast rule too.

☑ Never go hungry

☑ Plan your meals

☑ Keep a shopping list

Encourage family members to use it, too. If they need something, ask them to put it on the list. If you're in charge of the list you can vet their choices, which ensures nothing unhealthy enters the house.

☑ Keep your kitchen healthy

BOOK UP YOUR BUDDIES! The very act of talking about the things you are changing keeps these new habits at the forefront of your mind and will focus your attention on them, which is a really powerful way to ensure success. Better still, why not recruit some of your friends or family members to do The Accumulator™ with you? That's the goal for today. You can also join our established team online if you like, although all the information you will require is contained in this book. You can find the details at www.theaccumulator.net

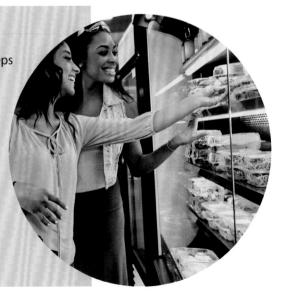

recruit
family
and
friends

DAY 12

Curb the caffeine

THERE ARE ACTUALLY **SOME PROVEN HEALTH BENEFITS LINKED WITH CAFFEINE. STUDIES** HAVE SHOWN IT CAN REDUCE THE RISK FROM TYPE 2 DIABETES, PARKINSON'S DISEASE AND EVEN SOME CANCERS. THE AMERICAN COLLEGE OF SPORTS MEDICINE HAS FOUND THAT CAFFEINE CAN HAVE A POSITIVE EFFECT ON PERFORMANCE WITH SOME EXERCISE. SO I DON'T SUGGEST YOU ELIMINATE IT COMPLETELY (IN FACT YOU SHOULDN'T BE *TOTALLY* ELIMINATING ANYTHING). TODAY, THOUGH, I WANT YOU TO SIMPLY EVALUATE HOW MUCH CAFFEINE YOU HAVE. I'VE COME ACROSS PEOPLE WHO REGULARLY CONSUME 10 OR MORE CUPS OF COFFEE PER DAY AND YOU WILL BE HARD-PUSHED TO FIND ANY RESEARCH THAT SAYS THAT MUCH IS GOOD FOR YOU.

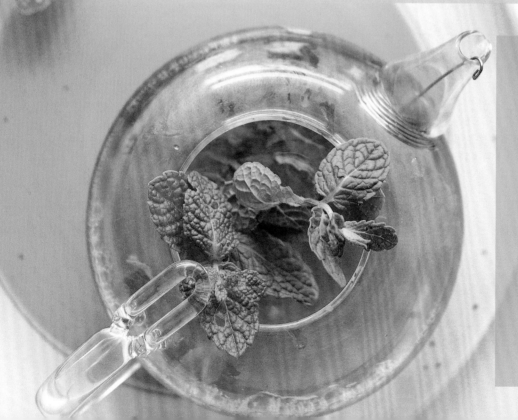

BECOME A COFFEE PURIST

Even though I'm saying a little caffeine is OK it does depend what type of caffeinated drink we're talking about. Caffeinated soft drinks and energy drinks are usually high in sugar too. As are many of the more fancy coffees you can buy in coffee shops. Try to take your tea or coffee as plain as you can. Black if at all possible. Try to avoid decaffeinated drinks too. They are usually made from a different type of bean which has been linked with a rise in cholesterol.

A quick recap

☑ Show your support

Have you found a healthy eating buddy yet? Make sure you continue to talk to others about your new regime and tell them how you're doing. Have you joined our team online yet (details at www.theaccumulator.net)? This is a great forum where you can chat to others who are experiencing the same thing as you, but your friends and family are also good choices.

☑ Practise smart eating

Eating out today? Make sure what you choose doesn't go against anything you have learned so far about healthy eating habits.

☑ Go nuts

☑ Go green

As we're talking about caffeine today, why not try some green or peppermint tea in place of your standard brew?

☑ Take the measure of your meals

☑ Break the fast

If you've kept this up, you'll be waking up hungry. If I have to go without breakfast in the morning, I'm a mess. I can't focus, I feel tired and all I can think about is the need to put something in my tummy. My body has adapted to expect breakfast, and yours should too.

☑ Never go hungry

The only time you should really feel hungry is first thing in the morning before breakfast. You may also still be experiencing those habit-related cravings, such as wanting something to eat when you're watching TV. If this is you, have a drink instead.

☑ Plan your meals

☑ Keep a shopping list

I'm lost without a shopping list and by now you should be too. If you haven't tried it before, grocery shopping online could save you time, money and most importantly, help to keep you organised.

☑ Keep your kitchen healthy

By now there really should be nothing but good, wholesome food in your fridge.

CUT BACK SLOWLY

I admit I love a cup of coffee, but I try to limit the amount I drink. A cup with breakfast for me is a must and perhaps one or two more at some other point during the day but, in general, all my other hot drinks are either peppermint or green tea. Count up how many caffeinated drinks you have today and if it's more than four, work to reduce this. Don't try to cut it down in one go though, just try reducing the amount by one cup per day until you hit a more sensible level and find something you enjoy to replace it. Remember caffeine has a diuretic effect so you just need to make sure you drink a little extra water to compensate.

switch cappuccino to
black coffee

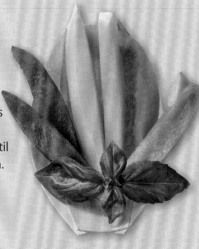

HIT THE FRUIT BOWL

When a coffee craving strikes try having a piece of fruit, some crudités or a small handful of nuts instead, until the habit is broken. Always carry some healthy snacks with you to avoid temptation.

DAY 13

Get some staples

I DON'T MEAN THE TYPE THAT YOU USE IN PAPER – I'M TALKING FOOD HERE. I'D LIKE YOU TO DO A LITTLE RESEARCH TODAY OR MAKE A LIST. I HAVE IN MY ARSENAL FIVE MEALS I FALL BACK ON IF I CAN'T THINK OF ANYTHING ELSE TO EAT. NONE OF THESE STAPLES IS COMPLICATED TO MAKE, AND HAVING A REPERTOIRE OF OLD FAITHFULS REALLY WORKS FOR ME AS OFTEN I FIND MYSELF WITH VERY LITTLE TIME TO MAKE ANYTHING TO EAT. TODAY, I WANT YOU TO WRITE A LIST OF FIVE STAPLES AND STICK IT TO YOUR FRIDGE (BUT NOT WITH A STAPLER). IT COULD EVEN BE SOMETHING AS EASY AS STEAMED FISH WITH SOME STIR-FRIED VEGETABLES OR AN OMELETTE. IN FACT, THE SIMPLER IT IS THE BETTER. MAKE SURE IT'S TASTY, THOUGH.

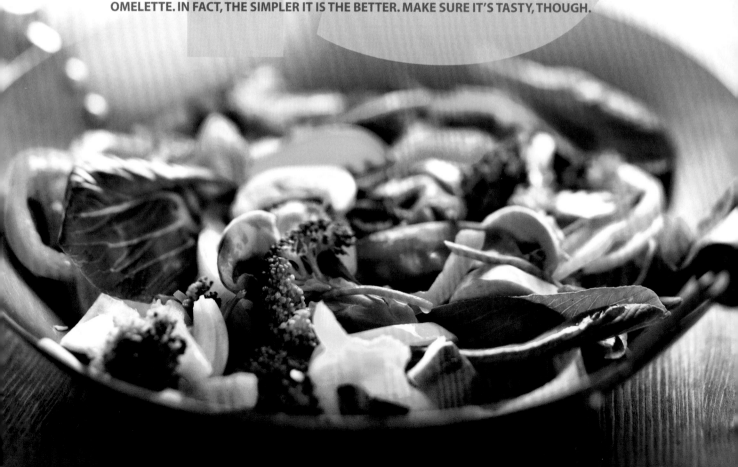

FEEL THE PULSE!

Take a look at your staple recipes and see if there are any changes you can make to pack an even greater nutrient punch. Can you add different vegetables, swap white rice for wholegrain or quinoa? Is there a good balance of macronutrients (see page 46)?

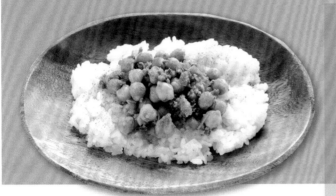

staple recipes and staple ingredients

STICK WITH YOUR STAPLES

Now that you've made your list of your five emergency meals, make sure you have everything in your kitchen at all times so you can make them.

ensure your staples are balanced

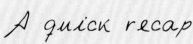

A quick recap

☑ **Curb the caffeine**

Remember to replace caffeine with water or herbal or fruit teas rather than decaffeinated drinks. Or how about hot water with a quarter of lemon?

☑ **Show your support**

Remember to tell your friends and family how you are getting on today and, if you're using The Accumulator™ online group, share your experiences with them too.

☑ **Practice smart eating**

If you're planning to eat out today you might want to use this as your treat meal. That's fine – just remember to keep to all your good new habits tomorrow.

☑ **Go nuts**

☑ **Go green**

Make sure that there is something green in all your staples.

☑ **Take the measure of your meals**

Adding nuts to a meal ensures you get an extra portion of protein and fat.

☑ **Break the fast**

You could even sprinkle some nuts on your breakfast.

☑ **Never go hungry**

☑ **Plan your meals**

This one should be second nature by now, but having a list of five fall-back meals will make it even easier if you run out of time or inspiration.

☑ **Keep a shopping list**

☑ **Keep your kitchen healthy**

Enough said. Ditch the junk.

DAY 14

It's treat day

ALWAYS TRY TO HAVE *ONE* OF THESE EACH WEEK. COMPLETELY DENYING YOURSELF THE FOODS YOU REALLY ENJOY WILL ULTIMATELY END IN DISASTER AS YOU MAY BEGIN TO CRAVE THEM. DON'T FORGET THIS IS ONE TREAT, SO DON'T GORGE YOURSELF ON AS MUCH JUNK FOOD AS YOU CAN CONSUME IN ONE DAY. BELIEVE ME, I HAVE HAD CLIENTS WHO TAKE THEIR TREAT DAY LITERALLY AND END UP UNDOING ALL THE GOOD THEY DID OVER THE WEEK IN JUST ONE DAY. SO LET YOUR HAIR DOWN A LITTLE BUT NOT SO MUCH THAT YOU TOTALLY FORGET ALL THE OTHER HABITS YOU'RE TRYING TO ESTABLISH.

A quick recap

☑ **Get some staples**

If you didn't complete your staple list yesterday, get it finished today. You may even find that by the end of the month your staple list will change. Remember, too, that this is a list to fall back on. The more creative you are when you have time, the more varied your diet will become and the more likely you are to get a good balance of all the vitamins and minerals your body needs. If you find yourself leaning on your staples list a little too much, you might want to consider putting more things on it. There are loads of great recipe ideas at www.theaccumulator.net.

☑ **Curb the caffeine**

If you don't drink much anyway, you don't have this habit to break in the first place. However, if you love tea or coffee, try to cut back slowly to no more than three cups per day.

☑ **Show your support**

Remember to maintain that accountability by sharing all your new habits with your friends, with the rest of the team online (if applicable) or by comparing your progress with everyone taking part with you.

☑ **Practise smart eating**

Plan for the meals you eat out as much as you now plan for the ones you have at home, and you can't go wrong. It is a good idea to look up a menu on a restaurant's website and choose what you will have before you go. That way, you won't be swayed by what your companions choose and succumb to impulse eating.

☑ **Go nuts**

☑ **Go green**

☑ **Take the measure of your meals**

Balance is everything. Remember, it's all about quality and not quantity and that applies to the variety of food as well as how unprocessed and fresh it is.

fruit share

GET FRUITY AT WORK! Try to encourage your colleagues at work to eat fruit. Take one healthy snack into work each day and ask your colleagues to do the same. Then, when you get to the office ask everyone to put their snack into a bowl. When it comes to that mid-morning or mid-afternoon break or you feel hungry, go to the bowl and take something that someone else brought in.

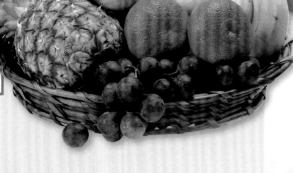

swap **ice cream** for **sorbet** as your treat

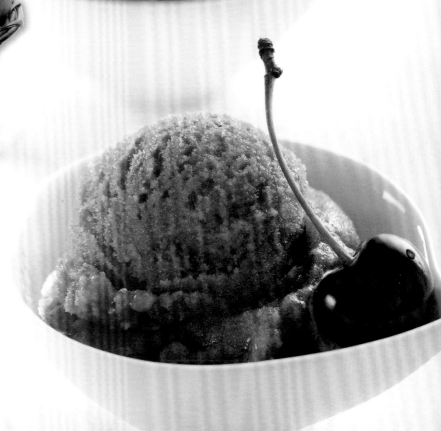

☑ *Break the fast*
I'll bet you can't live without it now.

☑ *Never go hungry*
A shared fruit bowl at work is a great way to avoid the vending machine and it also encourages your colleagues to adopt new habits and gets you to try some new snack ideas.

☑ *Plan your meals*
By now you're so good at this you've done it already, right?

☑ *Keep a shopping list*
If you're adopting the snack bowl idea at work, make sure you have what you need for your contribution each day on your list.

☑ *Keep your kitchen healthy*

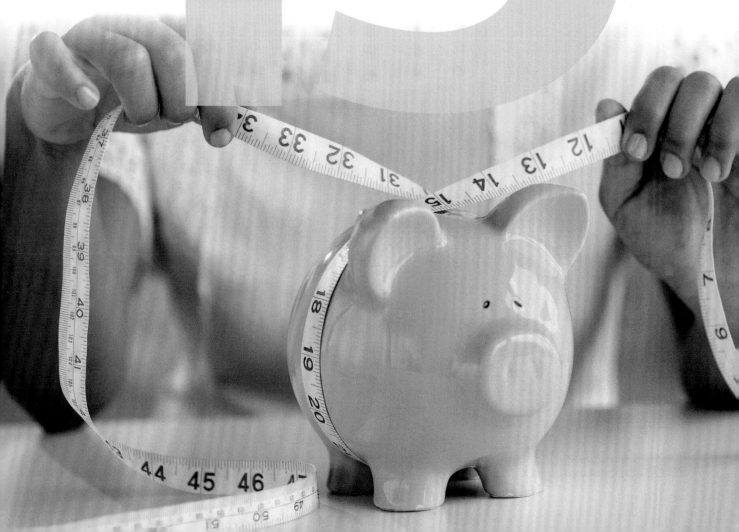

DAY 15

Give yourself a reward

THIS IS NOT ANOTHER TREAT DAY. INSTEAD, IT'S A METHOD THAT ENABLES YOU TO ACCUMULATE 'POINTS' THAT CAN BE ADDED UP AND SWAPPED FOR A REWARD ON ONE BIG TREAT DAY. THIS IS A GREAT HABIT TO GET INTO AS WE REACH THE HALFWAY STAGE, AND IT IS ESPECIALLY MOTIVATING IF YOU HAD AN ADDICTION TO SUGAR OR ANOTHER TREAT FOOD IN THE PAST.

IT'S NOT ABOUT THE MONEY...

From now on, every time you encounter and choose to resist temptation I want you to reward yourself. Think about the times when you pass a shop or newsstand that sells your favourite food. You might feel a little tempted but you keep walking. Or consider the days when someone brings in cakes or chocolate to hand out at work and you say no. Reward yourself each time by putting some money (perhaps the money you would have spent buying the resisted item) into a 'treat' box. Alternatively, put a slip of paper in there with an IOU for the same amount. Then at the end of the month, empty your box and treat yourself to something you really fancy using all the money you have saved. You may well find that you choose to buy a healthy treat, or perhaps some new sportswear, but if you do really want a piece of cake then that's fine too.

home-grown greens

are higher in nutrients

A quick recap

☑ **Get some staples**

By now you should have a list on display in your kitchen somewhere that shows five nutritious meals. If you see a great recipe or find yourself using one regularly, pin it up so that if you're stuck for an idea there's always something there to remind you.

☑ **Curb the caffeine**

Your shopping list should now feature tea and coffee less frequently and fruit tea or green tea more often. An added bonus of cutting down on tea and coffee is that if you take it with sugar, by drinking less you will also be reducing your sugar intake.

☑ **Show your support**

If you're using social media for this, make sure you've checked in and told the world about your new habit today (and mention the brilliant book you are using to do it, too …).

☑ **Practise smart eating**

☑ **Go nuts**

☑ **Go green**

If you have a garden, you might want to think about growing your own green foods. Start small with some herbs in a pot. It really isn't difficult to grow cut-and-come-again salad leaves such as rocket. Freshly picked home-grown vegetables are generally much higher in nutrients than those that have been flown across the world and then left hanging around on supermarket shelves – as well as tasting wonderful – so give it a go.

☑ **Take the measure of your meals**

Are you still getting the right amount of protein during the day? Have a think about all the sources of protein you ate yesterday – make a list. Was it enough?

☑ **Break the fast**

☑ **Never go hungry**

This should be automatic by now.

☑ **Plan your meals**

☑ **Keep a shopping list**

☑ **Keep your kitchen healthy**

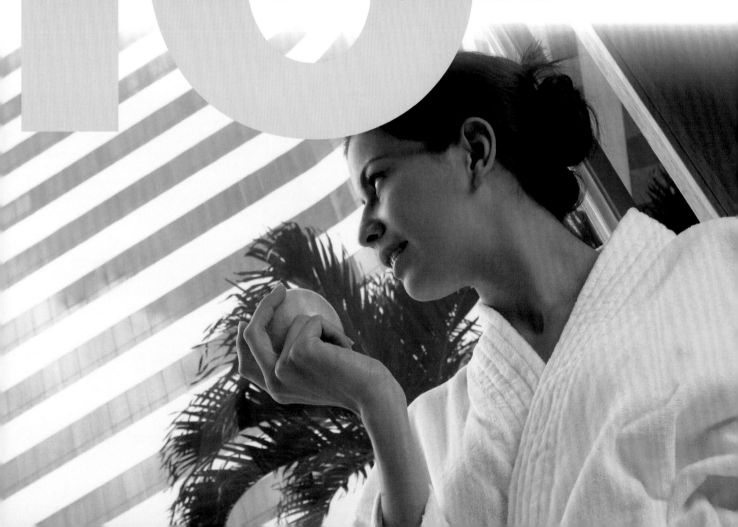

DAY 16

HABITS

Slow down

HOW MUCH TIME DO YOU ALLOW TO EAT YOUR FOOD? DO YOU SAVOUR EVERY MOUTHFUL OR DO YOU CLEAR YOUR PLATE LIKE IT'S THE LAST THING YOU WILL EVER EAT? I REMEMBER A FRIEND WHO USED TO JOIN MY WIFE AND ME REGULARLY FOR MEALS. HE ALWAYS, WITHOUT FAIL, FINISHED LONG BEFORE EITHER OF US AND EVEN THEN WE ALWAYS REMARKED THAT IT WASN'T GOOD FOR HIM. SO WE MADE A RULE THAT THE FIRST PERSON TO FINISH WAS THE PERSON WHO HAD TO DO THE DISHES; HE SOON SLOWED DOWN!

There are many studies that have shown that people who gobble are more likely to be overweight than slower eaters, because rushing your food can override the hormone that tells your brain when you're full. This means that you end up eating more than you would normally. So, if you think you're a fast eater, try to make sure you finish your meal at the same time or after those eating with you. Feel free to employ my washing-up trick if you have a family of fast eaters. If you're eating alone, try setting a stopwatch and aim to eat more slowly tomorrow than you did today.

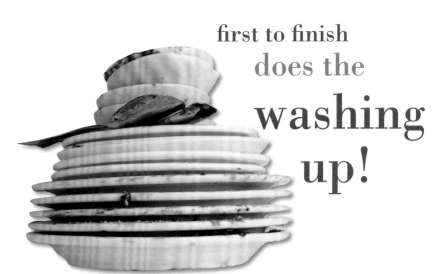

first to finish
does the
washing up!

A quick recap

☑ Give yourself a reward
Remember that treat box? How many times have you resisted temptation today? You may have even thought about what you might buy yourself as a reward at the end of the month.

☑ Get some staples
If you're sharing your experience with friends, you may well be telling them about all the new and exciting things you're eating as well as the exercises. Try to make today the day you swap some ideas and spice up your staples list with something new.

☑ Curb the caffeine
There are lots of hidden calories in some cups of coffee. For instance, a latte bought from a coffee shop can contain 150kcal or even more, and those laced with syrup, ice cream and other additions can contain twice that amount. Now, while I am in no way suggesting you start counting calories, be aware of the calorie content of drinks and perhaps choose a simple filter coffee with just a little milk if you like white coffee. If you take sugar, reduce the amount you add each time, until you have weaned yourself off it altogether.

☑ Show your support

☑ Practise smart eating

☑ Go nuts
Did you know that almonds are actually seeds? They're still really good for you though, so carry on eating them.

☑ Go green
Make sure your meals are colourful – not just green and especially not brown. If you have a plate containing foods that are different shades of brown, your plate will almost certainly be an unhealthy one. Eating a rainbow will ensure you are getting a wide range of different vitamins and minerals, as well as being pleasing to the eye.

☑ Take the measure of your meals

☑ Break the fast

☑ Never go hungry

☑ Plan your meals

☑ Keep a shopping list
I'll bet your current list looks very different from the ones you were making at the start of the month.

☑ Keep your kitchen healthy

DAY 17

Eat at the table

UNFORTUNATELY, DUE TO MY WORK PATTERNS I OFTEN STRUGGLE TO EAT WITH MY WIFE AND DAUGHTER DURING THE WEEK AS I'M USUALLY WITH CLIENTS AT THOSE TIMES. AT THE WEEKENDS, THEREFORE, WE MAKE SURE WE EAT TOGETHER AND SIT AT THE KITCHEN TABLE.

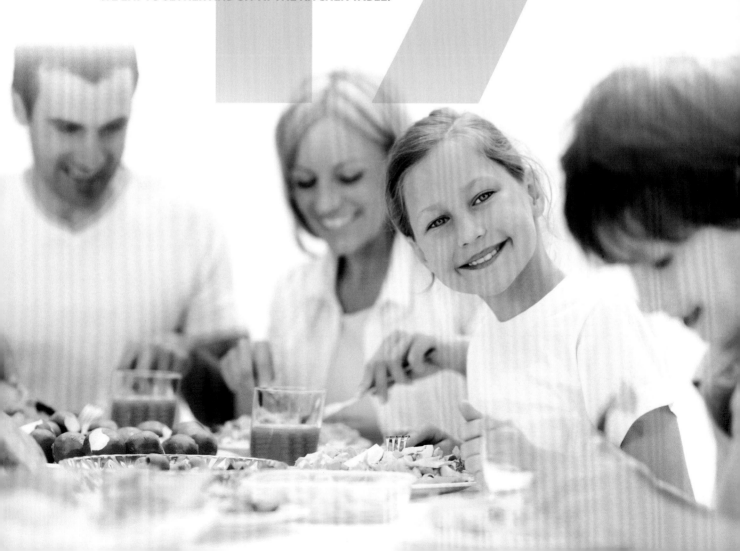

SIT DOWN AT A TABLE TO EAT Not only will this habit help to slow you down, it will make you much more mindful of what you are eating as you will be sharing the same food with the rest of your family. I also find this the best time to talk to my family as there's nothing to distract any of us. Well, apart from the food.

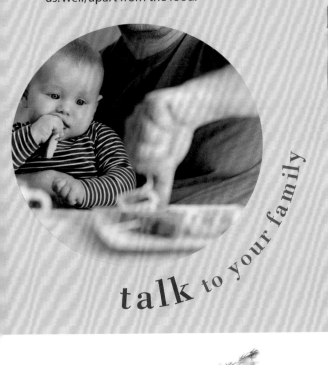

talk to your family

make your plate
full of colour

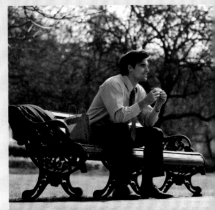

A quick recap

☑ **Slow down**
Make time for food. Whether you're eating alone or with company, ensure you have enough time to actually enjoy what you're eating. If you work in an office and the weather is good, why not take your lunch to the park? Eating outside in the sunshine will encourage you to take time over your food.

☑ **Give yourself a reward**
Did you resist temptation today? Put some money in the box.

☑ **Get some staples**
Do you know what your five staples are? When was the last time you ate one?

☑ **Curb the caffeine**

☑ **Show your support**
You should already have a group of people either following the plan with you or who at the very least know what you're up to. If they are regularly asking about your progress, you know that you're talking about it enough.

☑ **Practise smart eating**

☑ **Go nuts**

☑ **Go green**
Other colours are available. Make sure your plate is full of colour. When was the last time you ate something red?

☑ **Take the measure of your meals**

☑ **Break the fast**

☑ **Never go hungry**

☑ **Plan your meals**

☑ **Keep a shopping list**

☑ **Keep your kitchen healthy**

DAY 18

It's a naughty word

IF ANYONE ASKS, YOU'RE NOT ON A DIET. DON'T EVEN THINK OF THIS AS A DIET BECAUSE IT'S NOT. THE WORD 'DIET' HAS COME TO STAND FOR SOMETHING THAT'S TEMPORARY – SOMETHING PEOPLE DO SO THEY WILL LOOK GREAT IN A BIKINI ON THE BEACH OR TO FIT INTO A WEDDING DRESS. THE ACCUMULATOR™ HABITS ARE NOT ABOUT THAT. YOU ARE SIMPLY MAKING SOME PERMANENT CHANGES TO HELP YOU BECOME A MUCH HEALTHIER PERSON. MAKE SURE YOU NEVER SAY YOU ARE ON A DIET EVER AGAIN. THIS IS A NAUGHTY WORD AND DON'T USE IT (I AM ACTUALLY WAVING MY FINGER AT THIS POINT).

A quick recap

☑ **Eat at the table**

Gobbling your food in the living room in front of the TV is now banned. Mindlessly munching at your desk while still working is now a sin. Eating while reading, playing with your phone or doing something else is now illegal. Try to get out of the habit of doing anything other than actually eating at meal times. This will help you with the next habit.

☑ **Slow down**

Eating while you're doing something else will distract you from your food and may lead to you rushing or over-eating. So make time for meals and be mindful about what you are doing.

☑ **Give yourself a reward**

Pop some money in the box if you resisted temptation today. If you gave in to a craving, empty out all the cash from your treat box and put it in the nearest charity collection tin. Now start again with your treat box.

☑ **Get some staples**

How about finding one more to add to the list today? Or cook one of your staples but change just one ingredient and see what happens. Remember, there are plenty of good recipe ideas on the website (www.theaccumulator.net).

☑ **Curb the caffeine**

☑ **Show your support**

☑ **Practise smart eating**

If your're going out for a meal, take charge and choose the restaurant? That way you can pick somewhere that serves plenty of healthy options.

☑ **Go nuts**

Why not have a go at making your own nut butter or nut milk? It's really easy if you have a food processor, and it means you can eliminate any added sugar or salt.

☑ **Go green**

☑ **Take the measure of your meals**

☑ **Break the fast**

☑ **Never go hungry**

☑ **Plan your meals**

☑ **Keep a shopping list**

☑ **Keep your kitchen healthy**

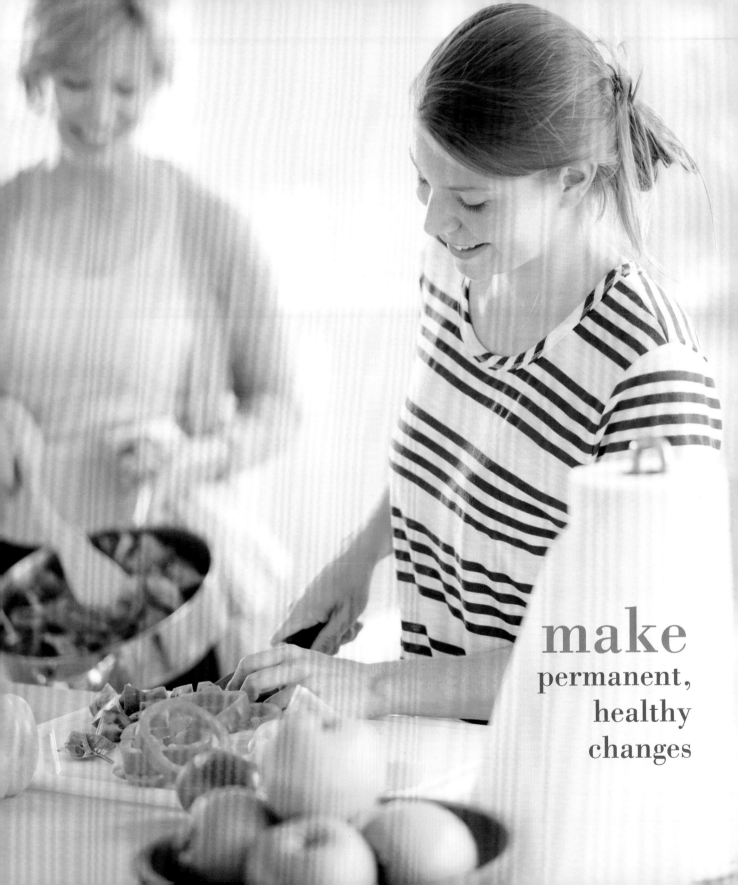

make
permanent,
healthy
changes

DAY 19

Get some sleep

THERE ARE SO MANY REASONS WHY GETTING ENOUGH SLEEP SHOULD BE A KEY PART OF YOUR PLAN TO BECOME THE HEALTHIEST YOU HAVE EVER BEEN. FOR STARTERS, SCRIMPING ON SLEEP CAN HAVE A DRAMATIC EFFECT ON THE WAY YOUR BODY PROCESSES FOOD. STRESS IS AN IMPORTANT FACTOR WHEN IT COMES TO BEING HEALTHY AND ANY EMOTIONAL OR PHYSICAL PRESSURE CAN CAUSE YOU TO HOLD ON TO BODY FAT. A CONSTANT LACK OF SLEEP CAN PUT A MASSIVE STRAIN ON YOUR BODY AND IN TURN CAN LEAVE YOU FEELING IRRITABLE AND MOODY FOR THE REST OF THE DAY. BEING IN A BAD MOOD CAN ALSO LEAD TO YOU MAKING BAD FOOD CHOICES AS YOU OPT TO COMFORT-EAT. SO, MAKE SURE YOU MAKE TIME FOR SLEEP.

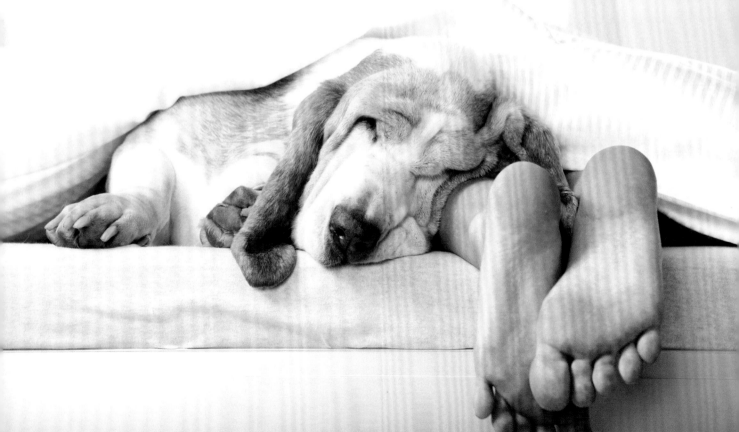

CONNECT WITH YOUR BODY CLOCK Aim to let your body wake up naturally at least twice each week. That means switching off the alarm and letting your body decide when it's time to wake up. On most weekdays, my alarm is set for 4.45 a.m. which means I try to hit the pillow by 9 or 10pm to get 7–8 hours of quality sleep. So believe me, by the time the weekend comes around I'm just about ready to throw the alarm clock out of the window.

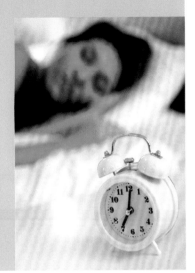

make a mealfie

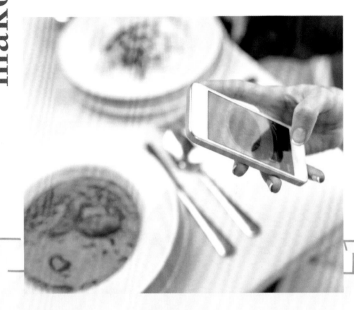

A quick recap

☑ **It's a naughty word**

Enough said. If anyone asks, you're not on one.

☑ **Eat at the table**

Try to make this a regular habit as much as possible. At the very least, make sure your mealtimes are either social events or ones without distraction.

☑ **Slow down**

☑ **Give yourself a reward**

You will probably find the times when you even think about temptation will now be few and far between, but they can still happen. Remember that reward when you say no.

☑ **Get some staples.**

Not sure what to eat? Check out your list. I usually have a chilli on mine purely because it's really easy to cook in bulk and freeze. This means I always have a nutritious meal in the freezer that can be ready to eat in minutes. Who says fast food has to be unhealthy?

☑ **Curb the caffeine**

☑ **Practise smart eating.**

☑ **Show your support**

Who did you speak to about all your great new habits today? 'Mealfies' (a picture of your plate of food rather than of you) are really popular on social media and are a great way to share ideas and maintain the impetus to eat healthily, since everyone can see if you are tucking into a load of junk food.

☑ **Go nuts**

☑ **Go green**

☑ **Take the measure of your meals**

☑ **Break the fast**

☑ **Never go hungry**

☑ **Plan your meals**

☑ **Keep a shopping list**

☑ **Keep your kitchen healthy**

DAY 20

Keep calm and carry on

THIS IS A PHRASE I SEE EVERYWHERE IN THE UK AND IT'S REALLY APPROPRIATE HERE, AS YOU WANT TO AVOID STRESS AND BE ABLE TO CARRY ON WITH THE ACCUMULATOR™ PLAN. STRESS IS REALLY BAD FOR YOUR WAISTLINE AS IT PROMOTES THE RELEASE OF A HORMONE CALLED CORTISOL. OVER TIME, THIS CAN CAUSE YOU TO STORE MORE FAT. IF YOU REGULARLY FIND YOURSELF IN STRESSFUL SITUATIONS, NOW IS THE TIME TO TAKE ACTION. HERE ARE 5 THINGS YOU CAN DO STRAIGHT AWAY THAT REALLY WORK TO KNOCK A STRESSFUL SITUATION ON THE HEAD.

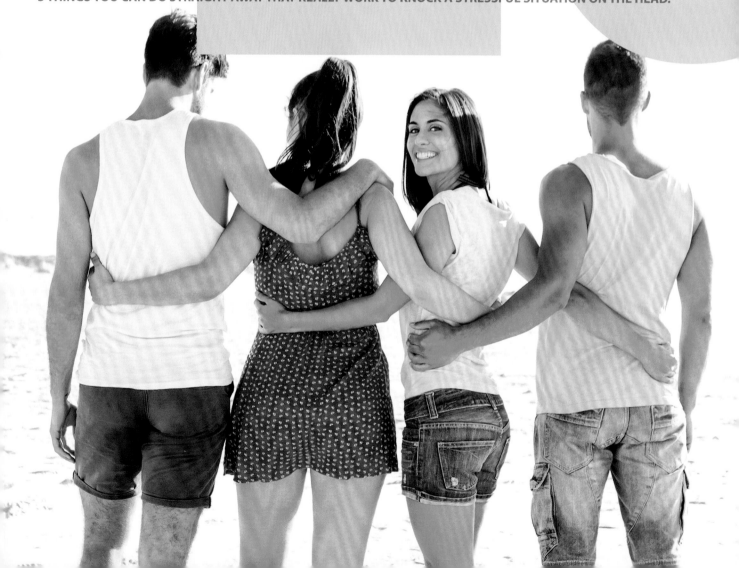

1

HUG SOMEONE I love a hug, and it's a great stress reliever. You don't want to be just stopping someone in the street here but if it's someone you've never hugged before, like a work colleague, it might be polite to ask first. The great thing about hugging is the more you do of it the more you get.

2

GET SOME SUNSHINE The sun is a proven stress reliever because it affects your levels of serotonin, a neurotransmitter that boosts good mood.

3

LISTEN TO SOME MUSIC Everyone has a song that instantly makes them smile. If you're stressed at work, nip out for five minutes and search for your favourite on the internet. Mr Blue Sky by ELO always does the trick for me.

4

DANCE Depends on how brave you are but this one really works. I remember doing this during a meeting once where things were getting particularly tense. I just stood up and went for it. Eventually most of the people in the room were dancing with me, no music, just dancing. The mood was not the same after that.

5

GIVE A COMPLIMENT Simple but effective. Making someone else feel good makes you feel good.

A quick recap

☑ **Get some sleep**

Listen to your body and don't fight tiredness if you can avoid it. If you find getting to sleep hard, try winding down to it. Try listening to some relaxing music. Even dimming the lights a little can be enough to prepare your body for sleep.

☑ **Eat at the table**

Remember to take time for food and avoid distractions. Clear away any clutter and turn off all devices before you sit down.

☑ **Slow down**

Eating is not a race. Make sure you have enough time for it.

☑ **Give yourself a reward**

☑ **Get some staples.**

☑ **Curb the caffeine**

☑ **Practise smart eating**

☑ **Show your support**

Remember, each new habit is as important as all the others that have come before, and while the ones you've been doing for some time are becoming really easy, you may still need to talk about the new ones to keep them at the front of your mind.

☑ **Go nuts**

☑ **Go green**

☑ **Take the measure of your meals**

Are you getting enough colour, protein, veggies, carbs and fat?

☑ **Break the fast**

Many people have exactly the same thing for breakfast every day. Ask the friends in your group what they eat and trade ideas.

☑ **Never go hungry**

☑ **Plan your meals**

☑ **Keep a shopping list**

☑ **Keep your kitchen healthy**

All the habits that you took up the first week of the plan should really be just that by now: habits. If you dropped one of these you would miss it.

It's a treat day

THIS IS YOUR THIRD TREAT DAY AND YOU SHOULD NOTICE SOMETHING DIFFERENT BY NOW. HAVE THE THINGS YOU ONCE REGARDED AS TREATS CHANGED? YOU ARE WELL INTO THE FIRST MONTH OF A NEW WAY OF EATING AND IF YOU WERE ONCE A SUGAR ADDICT YOU MAY BE AWARE THAT YOUR TASTE BUDS HAVE ALTERED. AS A RESULT, IF YOU ONCE WANTED SOMETHING SWEET YOU MAY NOT FEEL THE SAME NOW.

TREATS DON'T HAVE TO BE UNHEALTHY Personally, these days the only chocolate I can really eat is dark, containing as little sugar and as much cocoa as possible. For many this will taste much too bitter, but I love it. Dark chocolate in small quantities also has many proven nutritional benefits, such as helping to improve brain function and blood flow as well as triggering feel-good hormones. It's also full of antioxidants (which can slow down cell damage) and contains iron. So you see, my treat is still a pretty healthy choice. If you're not quite there yet, keep a close watch on this one – if you maintain all of the good eating habits, you will find your choice of treat will change.

your choice of treat will change

A quick recap

☑ **Keep calm and carry on**

Keep stress levels at bay and your waistline will thank you. Beating stress is a proven technique for losing body fat and it's no coincidence that exercise helps combat it too. Physical activity can cause the same chemical reaction in your brain as eating something sweet or even having sex. So, combining the healthy eating for life plan with The Accumulator™ workout described later in this book is a great way to overcome stress.

☑ **Get some sleep**

Don't burn the candle at both ends. If you have to get up early in the morning, try to go to bed early enough for you to get enough sleep.

☑ **It's a naughty word**

☑ **Eat at the table**

This habit is not really just about eating at the table. It's more about taking time for food and not allowing distractions to get in the way. If you have a table available, use it every day. If not, ensure you only eat at mealtimes and don't combine it with doing other things.

☑ **Slow down**

When I'm really busy I actually schedule food breaks in my diary so I don't have to eat on the go and therefore rush my food.

☑ **Give yourself a reward**

Did you resist temptation today? Remember you are saving for something nice and if you give in to that urge to have something unhealthy you will have to start saving again. If you're finding this habit a little hard, why not trust someone close with your money? Having support from another person will help to keep this habit working for you.

☑ **Get some staples**

☑ **Curb the caffeine**

Unless you began this month with a big caffeine habit, you won't actually miss those excess cups much at all by now. Don't forget it's not about eliminating caffeine altogether, as it's a good source of antioxidants and can actually benefit your fat-loss pursuits. In fact, I don't want you to eliminate anything; just change the balance of bad and good choices.

☑ **Show your support**

You should be talking about food all the time. You may even be a big influence on others and help them to adopt some of the good habits you've been getting used to this month. Share the love and that in turn will help to keep you on the straight and narrow.

☑ **Practise smart eating.**

☑ **Go nuts**

☑ **Go green**

Remember, nuts are a healthy snack as well as a great meal ingredient. If you vary what you do with nuts you will find it easy to include at least a few every day. The same applies to colourful veggies. A few slices of pepper can make a wonderful snack.

☑ **Take the measure of your meals**

You should be able to see at a glance by now if there's something important missing from your plate.

☑ **Break the fast**

I'm almost tempted to take this off the list by now because if you've been eating a healthy, balanced breakfast for the past 21 days you would really miss it if you didn't have it. However, if you're still finding breakfast a struggle, remember anything is better than nothing – as long as it's food and not a food product.

☑ **Never go hungry**
☑ **Plan your meals**
☑ **Keep a shopping list**
☑ **Keep your kitchen healthy**

These should all still be on your radar, so check them off. Don't go hungry, know what you're eating tomorrow, never impulse-buy when food shopping and keep the junk out of your house.

DAY 22

Pee
clearly

WE ALL KNOW WATER IS IMPORTANT. THE HUMAN BODY CAN SURVIVE FOR MUCH LONGER WITHOUT FOOD THAN IT CAN WITHOUT FLUIDS. WATER COMPRISES ABOUT 60 PER CENT OF THE HUMAN BODY AND IT'S REQUIRED BY EVERY LIVING CELL. WE NEED IT TO HELP MOVE OXYGEN AND NUTRIENTS AROUND; IT HELPS OUR BRAINS AND DIGESTIVE SYSTEMS TO WORK PROPERLY; AND IT PLAYS A PART IN TEMPERATURE REGULATION.

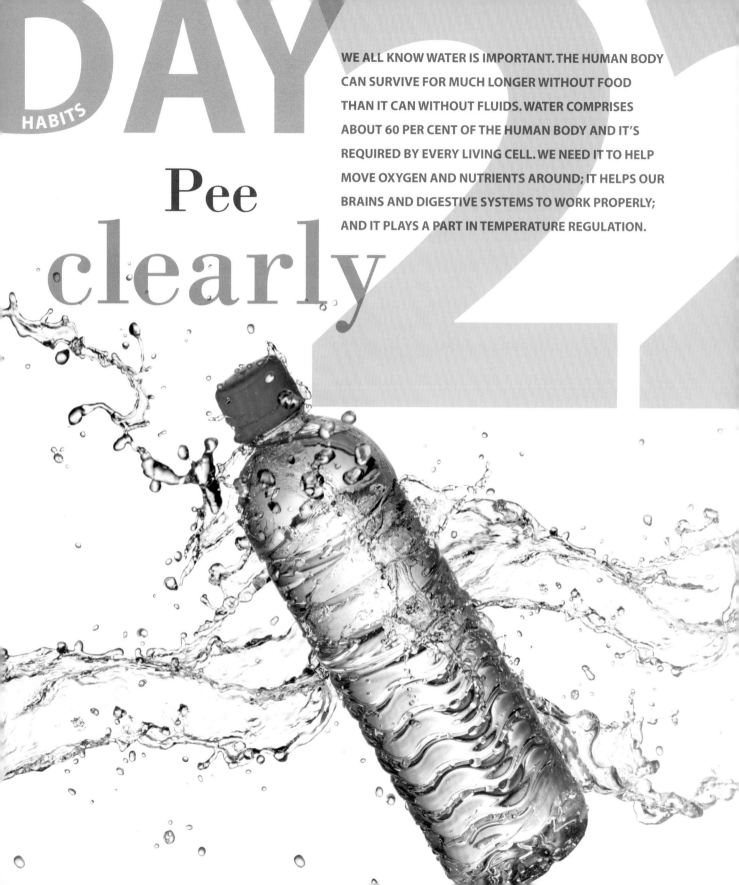

ARE YOU GETTING ENOUGH?

So the fact that many of us don't drink enough of it is crazy, right? But it's true. You might not even know how much *enough* is and if you look it up you'll probably find several answers. The popular volume is 1.5–2 litres (6⅓–8½ cups) per day and, while that may be about right, the exact quantity required by any given individual is dependent on many different factors, such as the amount they sweat, their age, gender, dietary habits, whether or not they smoke or drink, etc.

The best way to assess whether you are getting enough, or not, is to take a look at your urine. The more clear it is, the more hydrated you are. Remember, there is water in your food and not just your drink – an apple, for instance, is around 80 per cent water and a cucumber is 90 per cent water. So drink water, little and often, and make sure you have some with you at all times. Instead of obsessing about the actual volume you drink, however, check your urine to see how hydrated you really are.

IT'S NOT JUST WATER Other fluids count too, and there is some recent evidence that milk is more hydrating after a workout than water or sports drinks, since the fat in the milk lines the stomach and means your body doesn't just excrete it quickly; it absorbs more liquid instead. In addition, milk helps to repair muscles and can partially prevent DOMS, as well as being nutritious and filling. If you don't like water, try herbal teas or even just hot water and some grated ginger or a slice of lemon.

A quick recap

☑ **Keep calm and carry on**

Now you know how bad stress can be for your waistline it may seem almost ironic that so many people get stressed about losing weight. Bear in mind that you are working to change habits with this plan, not drop a stone in a week. Any change to your weight or shape will come as a result of adopting these new and better habits and if you have a lot of body fat to lose, it won't happen overnight. It didn't arrive overnight, so be patient. Permanent change takes time.

☑ **Get some sleep**

I want you to stop feeling tired. I'm not talking about the occasional yawn or the need to stretch – we all get that – but those moments when you feel so tired that you can't imagine taking another step or remaining upright for one moment longer. Your body will tell you when it's ready for sleep, and obeying that urge and sleeping well will help you to lose fat and grow muscle.

☑ **It's a naughty word**

☑ **Eat at the table**

☑ **Slow down**

☑ **Get some staples**

Remember to use your pinboard for inspiration when you find something new. There is an endless supply of really healthy recipes out there and now you can tell a good meal from a bad one you should be able to regularly try out new options.

☑ **Curb the caffeine**

☑ **Show your support**

From speaking to the people I have helped with new habits in the past, I find that they often become the support for their friends rather than the other way around. Stick to all your new habits and pretty soon people will be coming to you for tips and meal ideas.

☑ **Practise smart eating**

☑ **Go nuts**

☑ **Go green**

☑ **Take the measure of your meals**

☑ **Break the fast**

☑ **Never go hungry**

☑ **Plan your meals**

☑ **Keep a shopping list**

☑ **Keep your kitchen healthy**

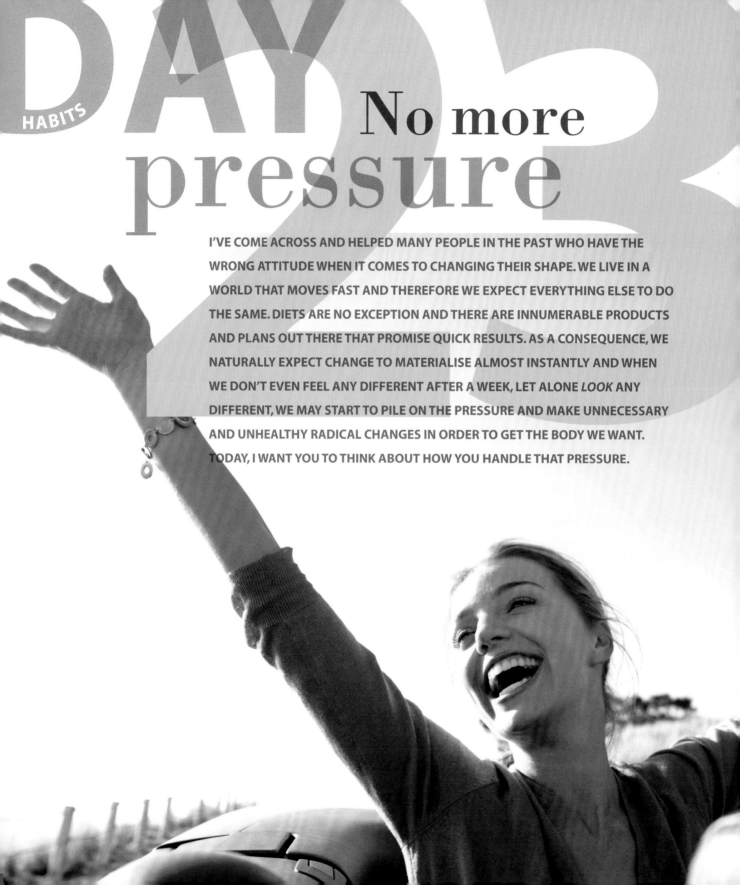

DAY 23

No more pressure

I'VE COME ACROSS AND HELPED MANY PEOPLE IN THE PAST WHO HAVE THE WRONG ATTITUDE WHEN IT COMES TO CHANGING THEIR SHAPE. WE LIVE IN A WORLD THAT MOVES FAST AND THEREFORE WE EXPECT EVERYTHING ELSE TO DO THE SAME. DIETS ARE NO EXCEPTION AND THERE ARE INNUMERABLE PRODUCTS AND PLANS OUT THERE THAT PROMISE QUICK RESULTS. AS A CONSEQUENCE, WE NATURALLY EXPECT CHANGE TO MATERIALISE ALMOST INSTANTLY AND WHEN WE DON'T EVEN FEEL ANY DIFFERENT AFTER A WEEK, LET ALONE *LOOK* ANY DIFFERENT, WE MAY START TO PILE ON THE PRESSURE AND MAKE UNNECESSARY AND UNHEALTHY RADICAL CHANGES IN ORDER TO GET THE BODY WE WANT. TODAY, I WANT YOU TO THINK ABOUT HOW YOU HANDLE THAT PRESSURE.

A quick recap

☑ **Pee clearly**

Remember, water is important. Is your urine closer to the colour of the water going in, or darker than honey?

☑ **Keep calm and carry on**

Many of us get worked up about the little things in life that at the time feel much bigger than they really are. Take a deep breath, tell yourself it doesn't really matter and smile.

☑ **Get some sleep**

Often we have trouble sleeping because we are stressed, and that lack of sleep can create pressure of its own. Spend 15–30 minutes winding down before going to sleep.

☑ **It's a naughty word**

☑ **Eat at the table**

Try to make mealtimes an appointment with either yourself or, better still, with your family.

☑ **Slow down**

How long did it take you to eat that? Could you have eaten it more slowly? Why not?

☑ **Give yourself a reward**

We're hurtling towards the end of the month. Do you know how you're going to reward yourself yet?

☑ **Get some staples.**

When was the last time you changed something on your staples list?

☑ **Curb the caffeine**

☑ **Show your support**

Many of the changes we established at the start of the month take no effort at all – you just do them and happily recommend them to your friends and family.

☑ **Practise smart eating.**

Remember you can enjoy yourself and eat out. You may even decide to use an important night out as your weekly treat.

☑ **Go nuts**

☑ **Go green**

By now a plate of brown food will look dull and unappetising and nuts will be a permanent part of your life.

☑ **Take the measure of your meals**

☑ **Break the fast**

☑ **Never go hungry**

☑ **Plan your meals**

☑ **Keep a shopping list**

☑ **Keep your kitchen healthy**

I've positioned this habit towards the end of the month because it's about now that you're probably thinking more about your results. Remember, this is not a short game – you're in this for the long haul. Only permanent change gets permanent results. You probably won't even notice some of the adaptations that are going on inside you. Switching to a healthy diet, eliminating the food products, removing your sugar addiction – all these things are causing the systems inside your body to work more effectively and therefore protect you from the long-term damage caused by conditions such as diabetes or heart disease. While you may not feel the benefits from making these changes immediately, you are investing in your future as well as your current health.

Don't put pressure on the outcome you expect in a few days. The further these new habits have taken you from what you were doing before you started, the greater the results you will achieve, both inside and outside. It's a good habit to just step back every now and again and consider why you are doing this. Think about the big picture.

DAY

Keep a diary

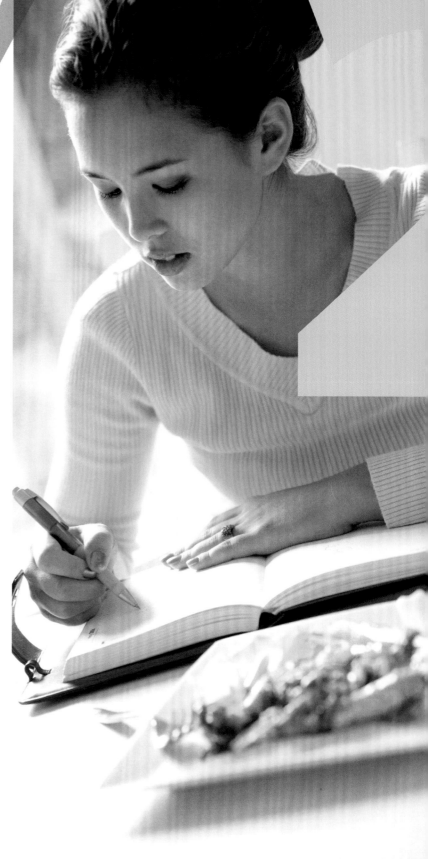

WHAT DID YOU EAT YESTERDAY? I MEAN EVERYTHING. CAN YOU REMEMBER? I'M GUESSING YOU'LL PROBABLY REMEMBER MOST THINGS BUT YOU WILL PROBABLY SKIP A FEW DETAILS. SO WRITE IT DOWN. THERE ARE TWO REASONS WHY A FOOD DIARY CAN BE USEFUL: FIRST, IF YOU'RE CONFIDENT THAT YOUR DIET IS THE VERY BEST IT CAN BE, A SNAPSHOT OF YOUR PERFECT DAY CAN PROVE A GOOD TEMPLATE IN CASE YOU RUN INTO TROUBLE IN THE FUTURE; SECOND, IT'S A GREAT WAKE-UP CALL IF PERHAPS YOU'RE NOT DOING AS WELL AS YOU COULD.

SEEING EVERY MORSEL THAT HAS PASSED YOUR LIPS WRITTEN DOWN IN BLACK AND WHITE REINFORCES ALL THE GOOD CHOICES AND HIGHLIGHTS THE NOT-SO-GOOD ONES. REMEMBER TOO, THIS IS NOT A CALORIE-COUNTING GAME, IT'S A QUALITY-MEASURING GAME.

A quick recap

☑ *No more pressure*

Try not to think of this as a diet and you will automatically reduce the pressure. You are simply creating some healthy eating habits that will contribute to a change in your shape and make you a healthier person inside and out.

☑ *Pee clearly*

Everything you eat contains some water, or it would be indigestible. A fish, for instance, is between 70 per cent and 80 per cent water. It all counts.

☑ *Keep calm and carry on*

Remember that stone I talked about earlier in the book? The one my daughter gave me that she found on the beach? Using something like that will really help you to keep calm and carry on. It will remind you of all that is good in your life and why you're doing this in the first place. Why do I exercise and eat good food? Because I want to be able to walk my daughter down the aisle, dance with her on her wedding day and play with her children. Not because I want to look good in jeans and a T-shirt. It doesn't have to be a stone, it could be anything small that reminds you of all the things that are truly important in your life and you are the most grateful for.

☑ *Get some sleep*

How are you feeling? Alive and full of energy or foggy and longing for the day to be over?

☑ *It's a naughty word*

☑ *Eat at the table*

☑ *Slow down*

☑ *Give yourself a reward*

You probably don't even think about all those foods that used to be hard to resist as you no longer feel the need to resist them. However, keep your eyes on the prize and remember to crack open your treat box at the end of the month.

☑ *Get some staples*

Your five fall-back meals should be changing all the time. Need some inspiration? Go back and look at what was on your list at the start of the month. You may even find you'll need to change one of the recipes as it no longer fits with your idea of a healthy meal.

☑ *Curb the caffeine*

☑ *Show your support*

☑ *Practise smart eating*

☑ *Go nuts*

☑ *Go green*

☑ *Take the measure of your meals*

☑ *Break the fast*

☑ *Never go hungry*

☑ *Plan your meals*

☑ *Keep a shopping list*

☑ *Keep your kitchen healthy*

DAY 25

Experiment

YOU KNOW BY NOW THAT SUPERMARKETS ARE FULL OF FOOD PRODUCTS THAT ARE REALLY NOT THAT GOOD FOR US. THERE ARE PLENTY OF HEALTHY CHOICES THERE TOO BUT YOU MAY HAVE TO HUNT FOR THEM, AS IT'S USUALLY THE JUNK FOOD THAT THEY PUT ON OFFER IN A PROMINENT POSITION. EVERY NOW AND AGAIN I POP SOMETHING I HAVEN'T TRIED BEFORE IN MY BASKET AND GIVE IT A GO, WHETHER IT IS SOME PHYSALIS (ALSO KNOWN AS CAPE GOOSEBERRIES) OR AN AFRICAN HORNED CUCUMBER. TODAY (OR THE NEXT TIME YOU GO SHOPPING), PICK UP SOMETHING YOU'VE NEVER TRIED BEFORE, THEN LOOK ON THE INTERNET AND FIND OUT WHAT TO DO WITH IT. WHY NOT TRY VISITING YOUR LOCAL FARM SHOP, ORGANIC SUPPLIER OR HEALTH FOOD STORE AND SEE WHAT DIFFERENT FOODS YOU CAN FIND THERE?

A quick recap

☑ Keep a diary

Did you write down everything you ate yesterday? If you did, you might find that you've made some changes today.

☑ No more pressure

Remember, it's not a diet. If you've only taken on board half of the habits outlined in this section, your body will be thanking you for it.

☑ Pee clearly

Drink it or eat it – just make sure you get some fluid on board and that your pee is clear.

☑ Get some sleep

Your body does the bulk of its repair work at night, so it's just as important as exercise.

☑ It's a naughty word

☑ Eat at the table

☑ Slow down

☑ Give yourself a reward

☑ Get some staples

If you picked up something new to eat today you might be thinking about what you can do with it? Do your homework, find a recipe or, if you can, try adding it to one of your favourite meals.

☑ Curb the caffeine

☑ Show your support

☑ Practise smart eating

☑ Go nuts

☑ Go green

☑ Keep calm and carry on

If you feel stress is still a big part of your life, use some techniques to help you manage it today. With practise, meditation can be really effective. Even spending 10 minutes listening to your favourite chilled music before bedtime could be enough to turn off the stress. Here's a really simple technique that I use from time to time.

1 **PICK A QUIET ROOM** where you won't be disturbed. Lie on your back on the floor or a bed.

2 **CLOSE YOUR EYES AND FOCUS** on your breathing. If a thought pops into your head divert your focus back to your breathing (this may take some practice). I like to picture a buoy gently floating in some water or a hot air balloon in a cloudless sky.

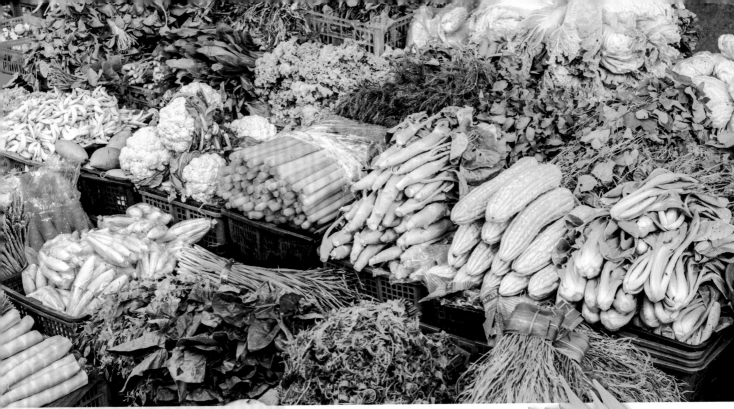

- ☑ Take the measure of your meals
- ☑ Break the fast
- ☑ Never go hungry
- ☑ Plan your meals
- ☑ Keep a shopping list
- ☑ Keep your kitchen healthy

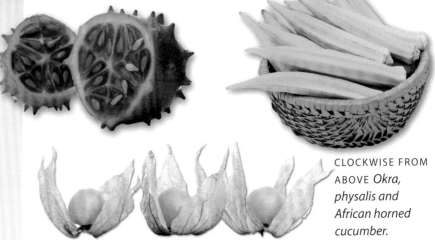

CLOCKWISE FROM ABOVE *Okra, physalis and African horned cucumber.*

STARTING WITH YOUR TOES concentrate on each part of your body. Tighten all the muscles in your toes and then allow them to completely relax – letting any tension disappear. Then move slowly up to your feet, calves, thighs and continue this process, one part at a time, through every part of your body. Take as long as you want to do this and try not to become distracted by other thoughts. If this happens, focus again on your breathing and continue.

3

WHEN YOU MOVE THROUGH YOUR WHOLE BODY focus on yourself as a whole and enjoy the feeling of calmness and relaxation. Focus again on your breathing before taking a big stretch through your whole body and opening your eyes.

4

Cook ahead

HOME MADE, BEST MADE This habit doesn't just have to apply to freezing either. If you know you're going to be in a rush in the morning, why not make breakfast and/or lunch the night before and put it in the fridge? Whenever I'm away for the day teaching or at a conference I always make sure I cook something that I can take and eat cold for lunch. I never rely on what may be on offer to eat when I get there as it can often be unhealthy (even at a fitness conference).

THIS IS A GREAT HABIT TO GET INTO AND IS REALLY OF BENEFIT WHEN TIME IS TIGHT. EACH TIME YOU PREPARE A MEAL, CONSIDER WHETHER YOU COULD COOK EXTRA AND FREEZE IT. I ALWAYS DO THIS WITH STIR-FRIES OR BOLOGNAISE AS THEY FREEZE REALLY WELL. THEN, WHEN LIFE IS VERY HECTIC I KNOW I HAVE A MEAL WAITING FOR ME IN THE FREEZER. IF YOU FIND TIME IS OFTEN AN ISSUE DURING THE WEEK, WHY NOT SPEND A FEW HOURS AT THE WEEKEND PREPARING SEVERAL MEALS THAT YOU CAN FREEZE?

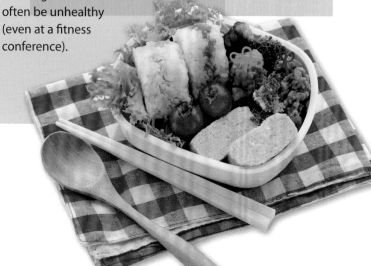

store meals in the freezer

A quick recap

☑ **Experiment**
Trying something new is a great way to educate and broaden your palate. Always make sure experimenting is on your radar even though you don't have to do it every day.

☑ **Keep a diary**

☑ **No more pressure**

☑ **Pee clearly**

☑ **Keep calm and carry on**
If the sun is shining, why not take your lunch outside or go for a walk? Being outside is a great stress-reliever and just a small amount of exposure to sunlight boosts your vitamin-D levels. Take care not to overdo it and burn, though.

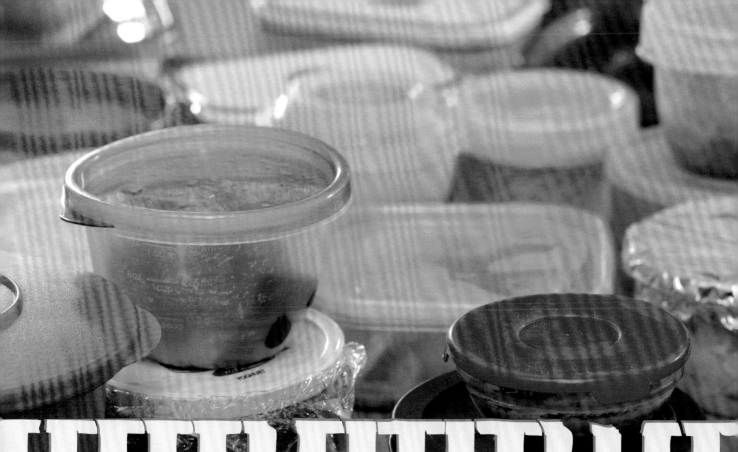

☑ **Get some sleep**

Don't forget to switch off the alarm clock when you don't need it. At least once per week, allow your body to wake up when it's ready to and not when your timetable say it has to. If you have small children, take it in turns with your partner to have a lie-in at the weekend.

☑ **It's a naughty word**

☑ **Eat at the table**

☑ **Slow down**

☑ **Give yourself a reward**

☑ **Get some staples**

Or freeze some staples. Can you make a batch of one of your five staple meals that you can freeze? Having a good back-up plan is a sure-fire way to make sure you don't fall foul of temptation.

☑ **Curb the caffeine**

☑ **Show your support**

☑ **Practise smart eating**

☑ **Go nuts**

☑ **Go green**

☑ **Take the measure of your meals**

☑ **Break the fast**

☑ **Never go hungry**

☑ **Plan your meals**

☑ **Keep a shopping list**

☑ **Keep your kitchen healthy**

DAY 27

Don't be a sweetie

WHEN WAS THE LAST TIME YOU ATE OR DRANK SOMETHING SWEET? I DON'T MEAN A PIECE OF FRUIT – I'M TALKING ABOUT SOMETHING PROCESSED SUCH AS CANDY, WHITE CHOCOLATE, A COOKIE, SODA OR EVEN A SLICE OF WHITE BREAD. IF THE ANSWER IS TWO WEEKS OR MORE, YOUR BODY WILL HAVE REPLACED MANY OF YOUR TASTE BUDS BY NOW, YOUR BRAIN WILL HAVE BEEN RE-PROGRAMMED AND THE SWEET TREATS YOU MAY ONCE HAVE ENJOYED WON'T TASTE THE SAME ANY MORE. SO TRY ONE TODAY AND SEE HOW YOU LIKE IT. YOU MAY BE SURPRISED THAT IT NOW SEEMS MUCH SWEETER THAN YOU REMEMBER, MAYBE EVEN TOO SWEET TO EAT. WHEN I WAS A FAR LESS HEALTHY INDIVIDUAL I WOULD EAT WHITE BREAD EVERY DAY – NOW I CAN ACTUALLY TASTE THE SUGAR IN IT. WHITE BREAD IS SWEET.

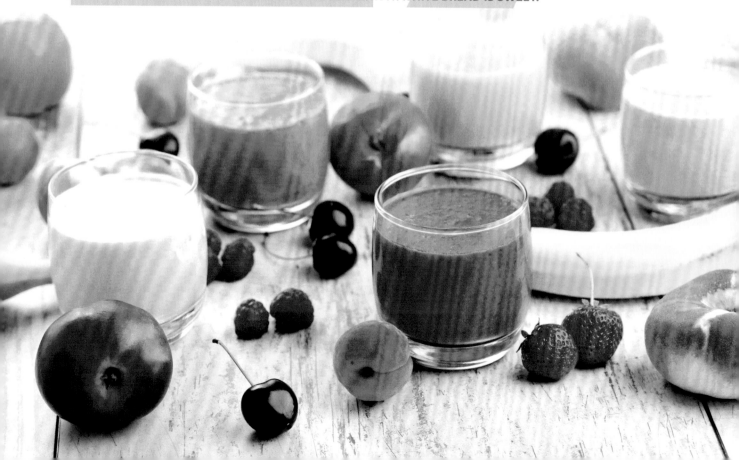

A quick recap

☑ **Cook ahead**

Do you have the opportunity to cook some extra portions today and put them away for a rainy day? Would preparing something today make your life easier and help you avoid eating something unhealthy later in the week?

☑ **Experiment**

If you're heading for the shops today or passing a food store you wouldn't normally visit, why not check it out and try something you've never tried before. How about some kohlrabi (right)? This vegetable is very popular in India and tastes great. Just don't be put off by the fact that it's an African word meaning 'ugly root'; looks aren't everything …

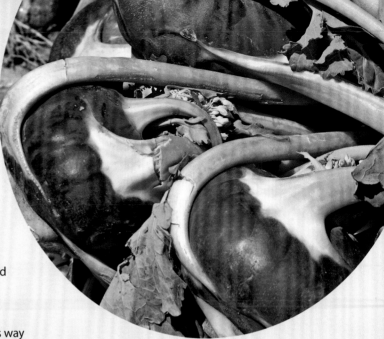

☑ **Keep a diary**

Remember to make a note of everything that made its way to your stomach today. Keeping a food diary isn't something you need to do every day for eternity. One week out of four is enough just to make sure you're eating all the right stuff and not slipping back into your old habits without even realising.

☑ **No more pressure**

Now you're coming close to the end of the first month of a brand new way of eating it's natural to expect some huge physical changes to have taken place. While this may be the case, you also need to be mindful of the fact that the majority of the positives are taking place inside you. Remember, this is a lifestyle transformation and not a diet – many of your results won't be measurable within 30 days.

☑ **Pee clearly**

How's the colour your urine colour today? Remember your first pee of the day should be the only one that has any real colour. If that's not the case, make sure you get some more fluid inside you (remember food counts too). If you feel as if you are properly hydrated there may be another reason that your urine is dark, and you may need to check it with a doctor.

☑ **Keep calm and carry on**

☑ **Get some sleep**

If you struggle to get off to sleep, try eating a handful of almonds every day. They contain magnesium, which will help your muscles to relax. Sleeping naked also helps. Really, it does. Your body regulates its temperature better when you sleep in the nude, and doing so also helps to increase your levels of cortisol and growth hormones, which means you will burn fat when you're sleeping.

☑ It's a naughty word

☑ Eat at the table

☑ Slow down

☑ Give yourself a reward

☑ Get some staples

☑ Curb the caffeine

☑ Show your support

☑ Practise smart eating

☑ Go nuts

☑ Go green

☑ Take the measure of your meals

☑ Break the fast

☑ Never go hungry

☑ Plan your meals

☑ Keep a shopping list

☑ Keep your kitchen healthy

89

TODAY IS YOUR FINAL TREAT DAY AND I WANT YOU TO REALLY REWARD YOURSELF. REMEMBER NOT TOO MUCH THOUGH. I ALSO WANT YOU TO THINK BACK TO WHAT YOU WERE EATING BEFORE DAY 1. BY NOW, YOUR DAILY FOOD INTAKE SHOULD LOOK VERY DIFFERENT FROM THE WAY IT DID AT THE BEGINNING.

DAY

Your
final treat
day

ERADICATE THE BAD Even if you were already doing some of the good habits we've been working on here, you will have undoubtedly managed to eradicate some bad ones and be feeling a lot better for it. Go back to those food photos you took before Day 1 (your bad mealfies). How much of the food you ate back then is still in your life today?

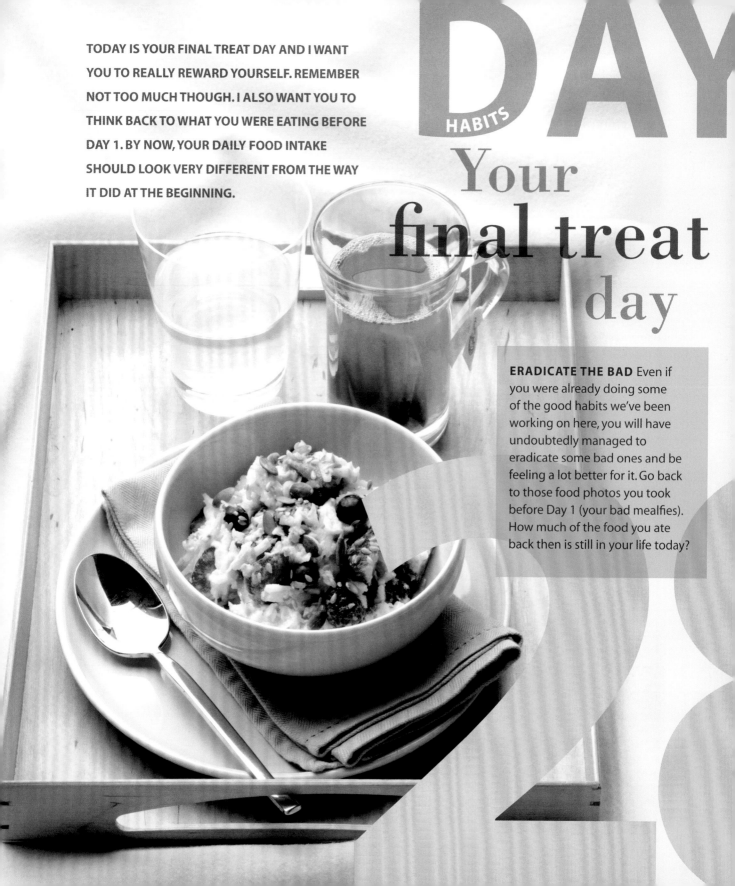

A quick recap

☑ Don't be a sweetie

Are you finding that you don't want to eat anything nearly as sweet as you did before Day 1?

☑ Cook ahead

☑ Experiment

What did you eat this week that you have never tried before? I remember my Grandpa having a bag of dried figs every Christmas and I thought they looked like the most revolting thing in the world (below). Many years later I decided to give them a go and now I can quite clearly see why he liked them.

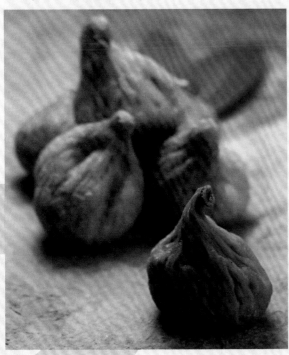

☑ Keep a diary

You don't have to write everything down – sometimes it's just easier to take some mealfies for a few days.

you feel better!

☑ No more pressure

There are only two more habits to add to your list and your new way of eating is complete. However, 'step off the pressure' doesn't mean you can think about slipping back to your old ways. The things you did 29 days ago are now in the past, and should remain there.

☑ Pee clearly

☑ Keep calm and carry on

Remember, laugh in the face of stress today. Whatever comes to try and tip you off balance is a mere blip in your life. Focus on the positive and not the negative.

☑ Get some sleep

Have you ditched your pyjamas? Did you ever think taking your clothes off could actually help you to burn fat?

☑ It's a naughty word

☑ Eat at the table

☑ Slow down

☑ Give yourself a reward

☑ Get some staples.

☑ Curb the caffeine

☑ Show your support

☑ Practise smart eating

☑ Go nuts

☑ Go green

☑ Take the measure of your meals

☑ Break the fast

☑ Never go hungry

☑ Plan your meals

☑ Keep a shopping list

☑ Keep your kitchen healthy

DAY 29

Go organic

IT MAY BE MORE EXPENSIVE, BUT IF YOU CAN, TRY TO REPLACE SOME OF YOUR STANDARD GROCERIES WITH ORGANIC ALTERNATIVES. FOOD THAT IS FREE FROM PESTICIDES AND OTHER CHEMICALS THAT AID THE GROWING PROCESS, OR ANTIBIOTICS AND SYNTHESISED HORMONES WILL OFTEN BE BETTER FOR YOUR BODY. THIS IN TURN CAN AFFECT THE QUALITY OF THE FOOD THAT'S ON YOUR PLATE. IF YOU HAVE THE ROOM TO GROW YOUR OWN VEGETABLES, THIS IS BY FAR THE BEST WAY TO EAT THEM.

GROW YOUR OWN I have only been converted to growing my own food since we moved to live on a farm, and I'm still amazed by the difference in taste and appearance between organic, home-grown vegetables and the ones you see in the supermarket.

CHOOSE ORGANIC If you can't afford to switch all of your diet to organic and for some reason can't grow your own vegetables, at the very least you should consider switching over to organic meat.

enjoy the difference

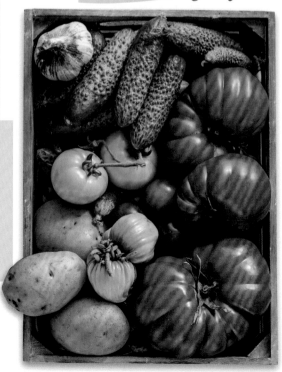

A quick recap

☑ Don't be a sweetie

But you don't really want to eat sweet stuff, do you?

☑ Cook ahead

☑ Experiment

☑ Keep a diary

☑ No more pressure

☑ Pee clearly

☑ Keep calm and carry on

☑ Get some sleep

☑ It's a naughty word

☑ Eat at the table

☑ Slow down

☑ Give yourself a reward

☑ Get some staples.

☑ Curb the caffeine

☑ Show your support

☑ Practise smart eating

☑ Go nuts

☑ Go green

☑ Take the measure of your meals

☑ Break the fast

☑ Never go hungry

☑ Plan your meals

☑ Keep a shopping list

☑ Keep your kitchen healthy

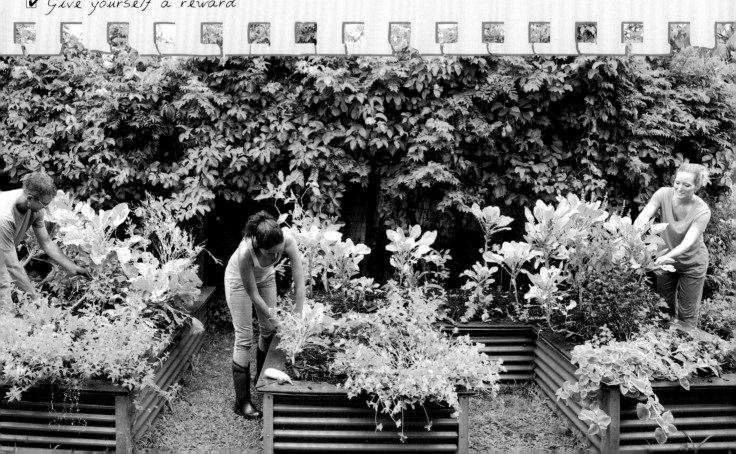

DAY 30

Measure your progress

WE'VE REACHED THE LAST DAY AND YOU'RE PROBABLY KEEN TO FIND OUT HOW YOUR BODY SHAPE HAS CHANGED OVER THE LAST 30 DAYS. IF YOU'VE BEEN TO A SLIMMING CLUB IN THE PAST OR DONE ANY KIND OF 'DIET', YOU MAY BE SURPRISED TO READ THAT I'VE LEFT THIS UNTIL THE END OF THE MONTH. WELL, A LOT CAN HAPPEN IN A MONTH AND IT MAY TAKE THAT LONG FOR SOME OF THESE NEW HABITS TO HAVE ANY EFFECT AT ALL. YOUR BODY SHAPE WILL NATURALLY FLUCTUATE OVER THE COURSE OF A MONTH ANYWAY FOR MANY REASONS, SO MEASURING YOUR PROGRESS MORE FREQUENTLY WILL OFTEN GIVE YOU INCONSISTENT AND POSSIBLY DISAPPOINTING RESULTS.

This plan is about much more than the image you see in the mirror – it's about internal health too, the stuff you can't see but will feel instead. If you've been consistent with every new habit in this book, you will probably be less bloated, and have more energy, better concentration and better, ahem, toilet habits. All these changes are as much a measure of your progress as what you see in the mirror. So today I want you to write down everything that's changed. Sure, measurements and appearance are important, but how do you feel?

There may be other things you will need to change to reach your own optimum health. For instance, many people find they feel better for limiting dairy in their diet or eating less red meat. The habits here are good ones for everyone to build upon, but bear in mind there may be more tweaks needed to really reach your own health zenith. If you feel there's still something not quite right I strongly recommend a session with a registered nutritional therapist as a worthwhile investment. Ask around your local area and see whom people recommend first, don't just pick the first one you find. You want an expert with a proven track record.

So now what, I hear you ask. Well, these habits are not intended to be adopted just for 30 days; they should be your routine for ever. To make it easier for you to remember them all (I haven't included the four treat days), I've listed them as a printable wall planner. A printable wall planner can be found at www.theaccumulator.net and www.bloomsbury.com.

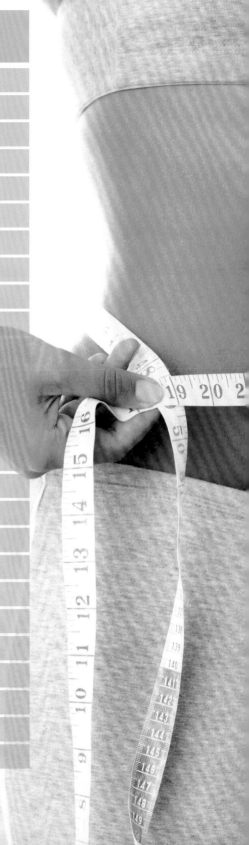

THE ACCUMULATOR™ HEALTHY HABITS WALL PLANNER

1	KEEP YOUR KITCHEN HEALTHY
2	KEEP A SHOPPING LIST
3	PLAN YOUR MEALS
4	NEVER GO HUNGRY
5	BREAK THE FAST
6	TAKE THE MEASURE OF YOUR MEALS
7	GO GREEN
8	GO NUTS
9	PRACTISE SMART EATING
10	SHOW YOUR SUPPORT
11	CURB THE CAFFEINE
12	GET SOME STAPLES
13	GIVE YOURSELF A REWARD
14	SLOW DOWN
15	EAT AT THE TABLE
16	IT'S A NAUGHTY WORD
17	GET SOME SLEEP
18	KEEP CALM AND CARRY ON
19	PEE CLEARLY
20	NO MORE PRESSURE
21	KEEP A DIARY
22	EXPERIMENT
23	COOK AHEAD
24	DON'T BE A SWEETIE
25	GO ORGANIC
26	MEASURE YOUR PROGRESS

B BEFORE YOU START THE ACCUMULATOR™ WORKOUT PLAN THERE ARE A FEW THINGS YOU SHOULD THINK ABOUT, ESPECIALLY IF YOU HAVEN'T DONE ANY STRUCTURED EXERCISE FOR A WHILE (OR MAYBE EVER). THIS CHAPTER CONTAINS SOME IMPORTANT INFORMATION. IN FACT, THESE ARE SOME OF THE FUNDAMENTALS THAT I MAKE SURE EVERYONE I COACH IS AWARE OF AND CONSIDERS BEFORE THEY START ANY NEW EXERCISE. EVEN IF YOU'VE BEEN EXERCISING FOR YEARS, YOU MAY NOT KNOW SOME OF THESE THINGS AND ADOPTING SOME OF THE HABITS HERE MAY BE THE DIFFERENCE BETWEEN SUCCESS AND FAILURE, OR EVEN INJURY.

Getting prepared

Get naked

Many people think this is a bit of an odd habit and I often get strange looks in the gym, but believe me it makes a huge difference to the way I train and it's something I insist my clients do as well. Now, let's get something straight before we go any further: by 'getting naked' I'm not suggesting nudity here. I would not suggest anyone do this workout with no clothes on, especially if you have company. You could have the most amazing body on the planet but nude jumping never looks good. All I'm suggesting you do is take off your shoes and socks and exercise in bare feet.

Now you may not think this is really all that important, but for the majority of our lives, our feet are the things that connect us with the ground. We stand on them, walk with them and run with them, but many of us have fairly weak feet and that's thanks in part to the things we put them in. Most people exercise in shoes that are designed to support the foot. They have thick soles that lift our heels higher than our toes and they squeeze our feet into unnatural shapes. All this supporting and squeezing can compromise the way we move. If you support any part of your body it will naturally become weaker. If you've ever broken a bone in the past and had it in a cast, you will know how weak the unused muscles become as they begin to waste away. When the bone is finally healed you need to work on the muscles to make them strong again. You wouldn't consider leaving the cast on for ever, would you? Shoes

act like casts on your feet, so by taking them off, your feet are free to move without restriction and you will develop better balance, stronger feet and an improvement in proprioception.

So what is proprioception? Many people regard it as our sixth sense. Close your eyes and touch your nose with your index finger. Go on, do it. What happened? You hit the target, didn't you. You didn't have sight, smell, taste or touch to help you with that, so how did you do it? Without thinking you instinctively knew where your nose was. Proprioception works with the help of receptors in your body that transmit information to your brain about the length and tension of muscles and the angles of joints. These receptors are incredibly sensitive and can detect even the slightest changes. A bare foot is capable of sending a much larger and more accurate stream of data to your brain than one that is covered in fabric and rubber.

When was the last time you walked barefoot on a pebbly beach? At first it probably felt very uncomfortable as the soles of your feet and your brain tried to work out what to do with the sensory overload it wasn't used to receiving. Spend a few hours on the same beach, however, and you won't feel uncomfortable anymore (unless the stones are very hot of course, in which case you should be wearing shoes). Your body has worked out how to balance and move on the surface. Try that with shoes on and you take a huge chunk of that sensory information away – you will have to rely much more on visual and auditory clues for your brain to work out where you are. Now translate that to exercise and you can begin to appreciate how much your movements can improve if your feet are naked.

There are a few things to consider when exercising in bare feet. The more of your day you spend with shoes or even just socks on, the more sensitive your bare feet will become. So, if you're not used to being barefoot, I would suggest you initially try it inside at home and then walking around in the garden before you even think about asking your feet to do anything more complex. Also consider where you are going to exercise. If you're used to getting your feet naked you may well be OK exercising barefoot outside, but might want to stay indoors if you are less confident. If you are going to follow this plan in a gym or other public space, check with the owners before kicking off your shoes. There are also certain conditions, such as diabetes, that can have an effect on the sensitivity of your feet. If you are unsure, it's always best to check with your doctor first.

Get outside

Remember you don't need anything more than yourself to do The Accumulator™, so why not take your workout outside? Obviously there are weather considerations to take into account, but if it's a nice day an outdoor workout has many benefits. For starters you will be soaking up all that vitamin D from the sun, and in addition exercising outdoors is a proven mood-enhancer and can help to reduce your stress levels. You can also up the intensity outside by exercising on uneven ground or even a slight gradient.

Make your feet stronger by spending time barefoot.

Get warm

As the workout becomes longer it will become increasingly important to make sure your body is warmed up before starting, especially if structured exercise is relatively new to you. Jumping into a workout of intense exercise from nothing can be a bit of a shock to your body and could end up causing you to run out of energy sooner or even injure yourself. A warm-up is essentially anything that will raise your heart rate and increase blood flow to the muscles you intend to use. Aim to spend around 5 minutes on a warm-up before starting The Accumulator™ each day. Try a combination of these exercises for up to 60 seconds with a 20 second rest before moving onto the next one. If 60 seconds is too long at first, start with 30 seconds and build this up as your fitness improves.

- Step up and back down on the first step of your stairs
- Run up the stairs and walk back down
- Skipping
- A run or brisk walk around up and down your garden or hallway
- Running on the spot
- Jump forward as far as you can, step back and repeat
- Squat and lift your arms above your head
- Squat as if you are about to sit in a chair and stand back up before you rest your weight on the seat
- Hopping
- Jump up and down on the spot

There are some warm up videos you can follow at www.theaccumulator.net.

Stairs are the perfect place to warm up.

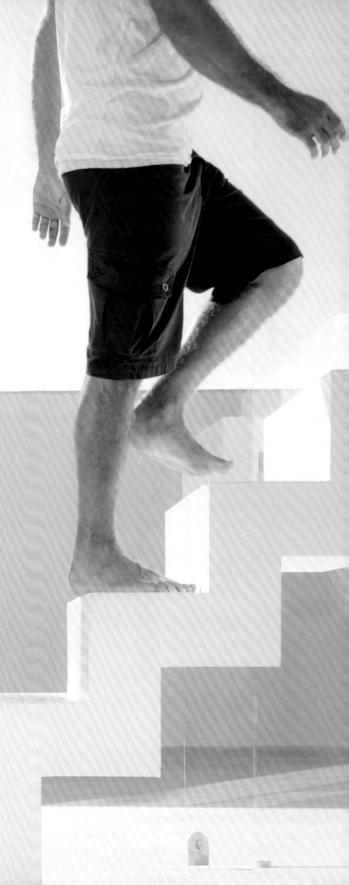

Get used to being uncomfortable

There are two types of pain associated with exercise: the good kind and the bad kind. The former is called Delayed Onset Muscle Soreness (DOMS); the latter is something a little more sinister and it's important to be aware of the difference between the two.

Whenever we ask our body to do something it's not used to we can expect to experience DOMS. Even if you haven't followed a structured exercise plan before, you will almost certainly have felt this sensation at some point after doing anything you may not be used to, such as going for a long walk or spending the day working in the garden.

So, here's what's going on when you get DOMS. Any activity that demands more from your muscles than they are accustomed to can cause microscopic tears to occur in your muscle fibres. That's OK though; don't panic because this has a couple of really big plus points. First, through this process your body is able to make itself stronger. You're laying down new tissue to make your muscles and connective tissue better equipped to cope with the activity in the future without going through the pain again. The other great thing about DOMS is that it burns energy. While your body is busy fixing itself it draws on your stores of glucose and fat to fuel the healing process.

The downside is that it hurts. You muscles will feel tight when you try to use them and may even be sore to touch. You might not even feel the DOMS at first until you try to use the muscles affected for an activity such as washing your hair, walking downstairs or even laughing. These effects usually come on between 24 and 72 hours after the activity that caused them and will usually take the same amount of time to fade away. Obviously their intensity and duration depends on how far away from your comfort zone you were when you exercised the muscles. If you get DOMS after The Accumulator™ workout, it's best to spend a day or two abstaining from rigorous exercise to give your body time to recover. Jumping back on The Accumulator™ wagon with a heavy dose of DOMS could result in injury and you don't want that. You can help to relieve your DOMS with some light exercise like going for a walk or a short bike ride. There is some evidence to prove that drinking milk can help reduce the aching from DOMS too. If your aches are a little milder, some stretching may help too.

You may also experience a burning pain in your muscles during exercise. This is usually as a result of the chemical process that goes on to make your muscles contract. The waste products produced by repeating the same action over and over don't get enough time to be flushed away properly and can accumulate, which causes a burning sensation. When you stop exercising this should fade away pretty quickly.

If you have any other form of pain during exercise or are in any way unsure about what you're feeling, it's best to stop and take a rest. If you experience any pain in your chest, or acute pain in your joints you should stop immediately. Stitches or muscle cramps can be quite common (especially if this is your first exercise for some time); however, if this or any other pain persists, stop and get it checked out to be sure there's nothing more sinister going on.

Muscles may feel sore the day after exercising.

Get your head right

Feeling dizzy or even sick during or after exercise is not something that affects everyone, but it can happen. Usually there are a couple of reasons for this:

EAT BEFORE YOU EXERCISE Your body needs fuel to help you move and will initially turn to glucose as a source of energy. If you haven't eaten for a while, or not eaten enough, you may not have enough glucose, which can lead to dizziness and may make you feel sick. This is quite common for people who try to exercise first thing in the morning before breakfast as they probably haven't eaten anything for 12 hours or more. Making sure you get some food inside you between two and four hours before you exercise can help, or you can try having something sweeter such as a piece of fruit (a banana is ideal) around an hour beforehand. Take a look at the section about the Glycaemic Index (see page 28) to help you better understand what's going on here and to help you make the right choices when it comes to your pre-workout food.

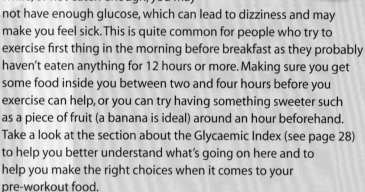

DON'T EAT TOO MUCH! Exercising after a meal can have a similar effect because your body is already busy breaking down all that food. Your blood is pumping to your muscles as you work out, leaving less available to help digest your dinner. Add in some jumping, squeezing and contracting and your stomach won't thank you for the whole experience.

If you find yourself repeatedly feeling dizzy or sick and you've tried changing your eating patterns, it may be worth turning down the intensity a notch or two (slow down). However, if it persists, there could be something else going on, which you need to get checked out by a doctor.

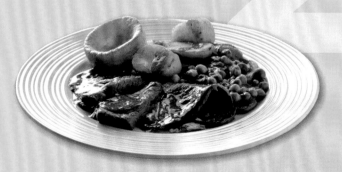

Should you exercise with a cold?

So you wake up in the morning, ready to exercise and you have a sore throat, achy joints and a temperature. Do you attempt the workout? Do you think, 'that's OK, I'll just go and sweat it out'? Or do you rest? This is one I get asked all the time. Should you continue to exercise when you don't feel well?

Exercise increases your body temperature, you burn fuel faster than normal, you lose water through perspiration, your respiratory and circulatory systems are stressed well beyond their usual levels, so putting your body through all that on top of trying to fight off a virus can put your body under incredible pressure.

If your temperature is already high, pushing it higher could be very dangerous. Keeping yourself well hydrated when fighting off a bug is important, so losing all that water through sweat can put you at risk of dehydration. On top of all that, you run the risk of injury due to a lack of concentration and increased fatigue. You will probably wind up feeling worse afterwards rather than better and it could take a few more days to get the bug out of your system as a result.

If you're still not sure whether to exercise or rest, try the neck check. If all of your symptoms are above the neck (sore throat, headache, stuffy nose), then you may be able to exercise but at a much lighter level than normal. Anything below the neck (aching muscles, nausea, hacking cough, diarrhoea) is risky and your body won't thank you for putting it through a workout. Nor will anyone else if you're doing it in the gym.

As a general rule, I don't exercise with a bad cold and if a client calls me feeling unwell, I generally tell them not to come and see me. You will recover much faster with rest than exercise.

How the Accumulator™ plan works

ON THE FOLLOWING PAGES YOU'LL FIND THE ACCUMULATOR™ WORKOUT PLAN. FROM START TO FINISH THE REGIME WILL LAST FOR 30 DAYS. DURING THAT TIME YOU'LL BE EXERCISING FOR 26 OF THOSE DAYS AND RESTING FOR FOUR. AS I'VE MENTIONED PREVIOUSLY, IF YOU HAVE TO TAKE A FEW UNSCHEDULED REST DAYS ALONG THE WAY TO COPE WITH DOMS, THAT'S OK. HOWEVER, YOU SHOULD AIM TO FINISH THE PLAN BY DAY 35 AT THE VERY MOST.

On each page you'll find photos along with a detailed description of each exercise. In many cases you will see two versions of the same exercise, one more advanced than the other. There are also explanations of how each exercise can be useful in your everyday life or how it relates to a certain sport or activity. Many of the exercises in The Accumulator™ are there to help you live a better and more active life, and it's useful to understand why you're doing them.

This is important because if you're not feeling it in the right places you may be doing something wrong. Even something as trivial as the position of your feet could change how the exercise affects your body. Bear in mind as the workout progresses you will be doing other exercises before and afterwards, which will mean you will be using the same muscles repeatedly. This can have a cumulative effect on the way it makes your body feel.

On your first day, do the exercise on the page titled Day 1. On the second day, turn the page and do the exercise on the page titled Day 2 then go back and repeat Day 1. By the end of the plan you'll be doing the exercise on the page titled Day 30, then working back through the book until you get back to Day 1. On each page you'll find a list of the exercises for that day, so if you need a reminder you won't have to keep turning pages (although that would be great exercise for your fingers). I suggest you rest on Days 6, 12, 18 and 24. As you work through the book I'll remind you when these rest days come up.

WATCH THE CLOCK

Rather than measuring your workout with repetitions of each movement, The Accumulator™ works on time. The first time you work through the whole 30 days I would suggest following this structure:

Exercise: 20 seconds
Rest: 10 seconds
Repeat the exercise: 20 seconds
Rest: 20 seconds
Move on to next exercise

If you follow this structure each day, by the time you get to Day 5, for example, your workout should pan out like this.

Russian twist:
- 20 seconds' work
- 10 seconds' rest
- 20 seconds' work
- 20 seconds' rest

Press-up:
- 20 seconds' work
- 10 seconds' rest
- 20 seconds' work
- 20 seconds' rest

Deadlift:
- 20 seconds' work
- 10 seconds' rest
- 20 seconds' work
- 20 seconds' rest

Twisted side lunge:
- 20 seconds' work
- 10 seconds' rest
- 20 seconds' work
- 20 seconds' rest

Squat:
- 20 seconds' work
- 10 seconds' rest
- 20 seconds' work
- 20 seconds' rest

Read this if you don't normally exercise or are returning after a long break

The plan starts slowly. Really slowly. In fact on Day 1 you only have to do one exercise for a total of 40 seconds with a 10-second break in the middle. Now there's a really good reason for this. If you haven't done any structured activity for some time (maybe even several years) the mere thought of spending 30 minutes or more building up a sweat and becoming uncomfortable can be very scary. In fact, for many the prospect is so alarming that it never becomes anything more than just a thought. However, those of us who exercise regularly know it has many benefits and the most important one here is that it makes you feel good, and that feeling can become addictive. I want you to become hooked, enjoy The Accumulator™ and not be scared of it. I know how good it will be for you.

Remember, on Day 1 you are only going to exercise for 40 seconds – less time than it takes to boil a kettle. In fact, you can do it while you boil the kettle. Everybody can do that. Chances are you do more exercise over the course of a day than that anyway. Even by the end of Week 1 you'll still only be exercising for a total of four minutes and with all the rest periods the whole workout by the end of that week only takes eight minutes.

As The Accumulator™ workout gets longer and the days progress, you will start to enjoy that special type of satisfaction you get from exercise. Other big advantages to be gained from adopting The Accumulator™ workout plan include the fact that you will become better at the exercises because you are doing them almost every day. The exercise you start with on Day 1 will still be performed on Day 30; by that time you will have done your first exercise for 25 days, so you should be pretty good at it. Many people also find that they can progress from the easier to the more advanced version of some exercises before they reach the end of the month.

The Accumulator™ is also a challenge. As you start to enjoy the benefits of regular exercise it will become a personal test you set yourself each day. This brings with it a great level of self-satisfaction, which also helps to make you feel good. The Accumulator™ team regularly contribute to a group on Facebook (which you are welcome to join) and often can't wait to tell the other members when they have completed each day and share how they got on.

RIGHT *Long jump p173*
BELOW *Squat p110*

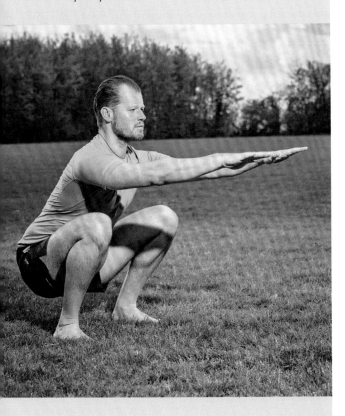

Read this if you already regularly exercise

If you already have a regular exercise habit, you might think that the first week of this workout plan is a little bit tame. Initially you may want to incorporate it into your current routine, whatever that may be. However, as the plan progresses into Week 2 you may be surprised by how challenging it can become. Depending on your current level of fitness, you may want to start cutting back on your existing routine so you can devote more of your energy to The Accumulator™ workout.

When I first came up with The Accumulator™, I only intended it to last for one month. As soon as that first month came to a close the people who took part were hungry for another, so I started rolling out new monthly plans. I discovered that starting again on Day 1 with only 40 seconds of exercise has a number of benefits. For the first-timer, there are obvious advantages to starting slowly. However, for those people who took part the previous month, going from the more intense, challenging final week of one month into the much easier beginning of another one actually gave their body time to recover and they were refreshed and ready to go as the plan grew in intensity again. Recovery is a vital component of any fitness plan as it allows your body time to repair and grow stronger.

What to do beyond Day 30

Once you've worked through the whole month don't simply go back to the beginning and start again. Constantly repeating the same workout is a mistake I see people making all the time when they exercise. As you become stronger there are many changes that take place inside you, and your body thrives on change. Your brain and muscles very quickly adapt to anything new and once you become efficient at a certain exercise your body will no longer be stimulated to change further. In addition, things will pretty quickly become boring, you'll hit a plateau and may even consider giving up.

There is a number of ways to adapt The Accumulator™ workout plan given in this book so it becomes different enough to make it a challenge all over again the next month. With The Accumulator™, it's not just each individual exercise that makes the workout a test; it's also the combination of exercises that have an impact. Simply changing one element, such as the order, duration or intensity can have a dramatic effect. At the back of this book there are several examples you can try beyond Day 30 to dial things up.

RIGHT *Sit out p165*

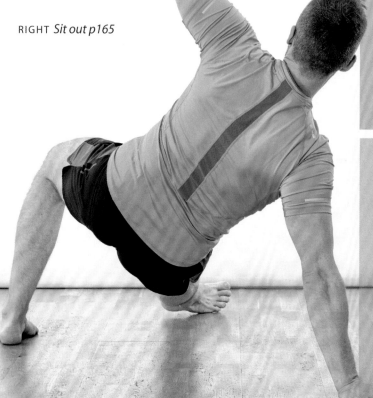

SHOULD I DO THE EASY OR MORE ADVANCED EXERCISES?

Many of the exercises have easier or more advanced versions. If you can't perform the advanced one safely with correct technique for the whole 20 seconds, don't. Go for the easier option to begin with, then once you feel ready you can attempt the tougher version.

FAST OR SLOW?

Technique is much more important than the number of repetitions you can do within the 20 seconds. If you can perform the exercise correctly and maintain speed then do so, but make sure your form is 100 per cent correct first. Start slowly, performing fewer repetitions within the 20 seconds until you are confident that you can up the speed without compromising on technique.

DO I HAVE TO DO IT EVERY DAY?

Ideally, yes. The Accumulator™ workout plan is designed to help your fitness improve, so you will need to set time aside to do this each day. There are four rest days built into the plan to help your body recover but you can always use these to catch up if you miss a day earlier that week. By the end of the month you will need to set aside around 30 minutes per day to complete the whole workout.

WHAT TIME OF THE DAY SHOULD I DO THE EXERCISES?

This is really dependent on you and your lifestyle. Some people have the flexibility to choose the best time for them, others may be restricted by work, children or other factors. Try to avoid accumulating late in the evening before you go to bed, however, as this could affect the quality of your sleep. I would suggest you experiment, find the best time for you and then put it in your diary. One of the many great things about The Accumulator™ is that it doesn't take long to do, so you should find it easy to fit in at some point.

All about HIIT

THE EXERCISE PART OF THE ACCUMULATOR™ DELIVERS RESULTS IN A VERY SHORT SPACE OF TIME. THIS EFFICIENCY IS LARGELY DOWN TO THE TYPES OF EXERCISES PERFORMED IN THE WORKOUT AND THE ORDER IN WHICH THEY APPEAR. THE FORMAT WORKS USING SHORT BURSTS OF INTENSE EXERCISE RATHER THAN A SERIES OF REPETITIONS. THIS METHOD OF EXERCISE IS KNOWN AS HIGH INTENSITY INTERVAL TRAINING (HIIT). IT'S A PHRASE YOU MAY HAVE HEARD IN THE MEDIA OR SEEN IN YOUR LOCAL GYM.

At the time of writing, HIIT workouts are very popular and there are myriad books, DVDs and workouts on the market that claim it is the latest thing. The Accumulator™ uses this system because it works and because it's been a tried-and-tested method of exercise that's been in existence for as long as we have.

There are no hard-and-fast rules to HIIT, but essentially it's defined as repeated brief sessions of intense work separated by intervals of lower-intensity work or rest. This is a method of exercising that we do all the time without even realising,

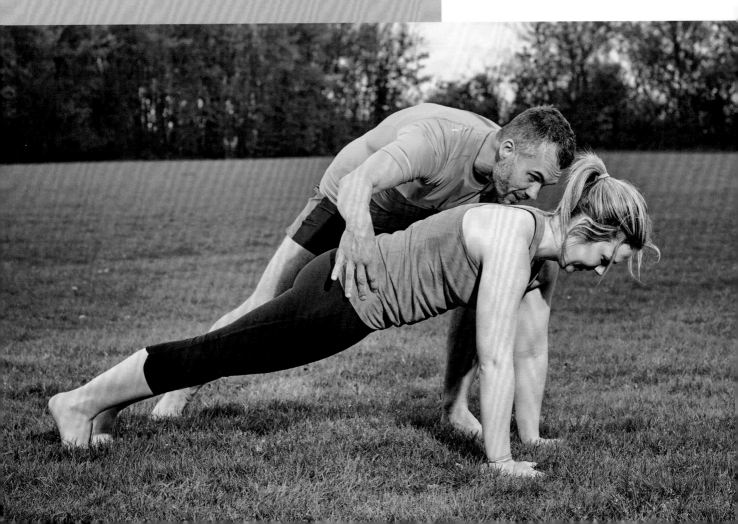

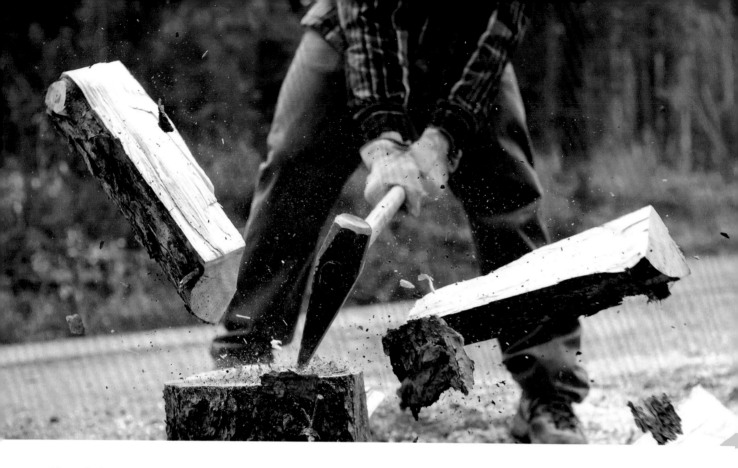

although the increase in gadgets and labour-saving devices means that we do less of it now than we used to.

Using HIIT in everyday life

As I have mentioned previously, I live on a farm and every winter I enjoy sitting in front of the log burner in our lounge. This does mean I need logs and rather than have someone deliver a truck-load every year I get a certain amount of primal, masculine pleasure from collecting and chopping up my own. Whenever I hear of someone in my village chopping down or re-shaping a tree I go and ask if I can have the logs that are littering their garden. Usually my offer of taking them away is greeted with a smile (unless my next-door neighbour gets there first). If you've ever spent a few hours chopping up firewood you'll know that unless you opt for a labour-saving chainsaw it can be very hard

work – a proper workout. You can only keep at it for a short period of time until you are too tired to carry on. Then, after a short rest you recover sufficiently to try again. Many years ago people used wood as their main source of fuel and a session outside cutting up logs by hand for winter was a regular activity. Well, chopping up wood is just like HIIT.

There is much evidence that our primal ancestors once used a form of HIIT in order to hunt, running for many miles to chase down an animal for dinner. This often involved short bursts of more intense running together with lighter, slower movements, especially as we drew closer to our intended victim. We know this because there are numerous tribes across the planet that still use a similar technique to hunt today. In the Western world, we channel this activity into organised games, and lots of sports are actually HIIT in disguise. Take football, for instance: short bursts of intense activity when the ball gets closer to you followed by longer bursts of less rigorous action. This method of exercise is so natural that we do it as children without even knowing it.

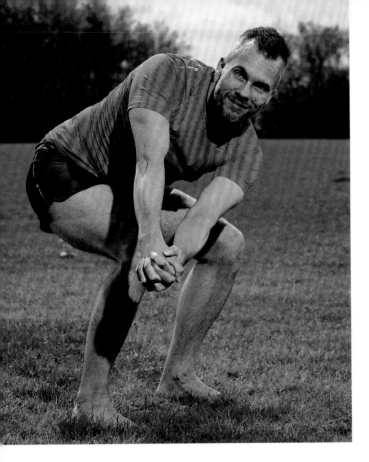

LEFT AND FAR LEFT *The Accumulator™ is built around movements we make every day.*

How is HIIT of benefit?

There has been much research and many studies published over recent years about HIIT and its benefits. One of the well-known ones was conducted in 1996 by Dr. Izumi Tabata from the National Institute of Fitness and Sports in Tokyo. It's his name that has since been adopted by many classes worldwide. His study used highly trained athletes and they performed intense exercise for 20 seconds followed by 10 seconds of rest. They did this non-stop for four minutes. He compared this with steady state training (exercising at a constant lower level of intensity for longer periods) and found that the more intense methods of training were of much greater benefit in a shorter space of time.

So why is HIIT so good for us? One of the biggest benefits of HIIT and the reason why it's so popular is something called Excess Post-exercise Oxygen Consumption (EPOC). Essentially, this is the scientific way of saying that your oxygen consumption remains elevated for as much as 48 hours after the exercise has finished. This is nothing new either (an English physiologist called Archibald Hill was looking into the phenomenon in 1922). All exercise burns energy while we are doing it, but high-intensity exercise continues to burn energy for some time afterwards too as we recover and our body adapts to the increase in activity. This can carry on for a day or more and the research shows that much of the energy we use to fuel this recovery process comes from our fat stores.

Because HIIT can deliver greater results in a shorter space of time, the technique also takes care of the most common excuse for not exercising: a lack of time. This isn't a laziness issue either – it doesn't seem to matter how old we are, how fit we are, what gender we are or where we live, not having enough time is the biggest reason why many of us don't do any kind of regular exercise

So if HIIT really does give you the best, fastest results, there really is no excuse for not exercising, is there? But let's face it, given the choice between relaxing in front of the TV and jumping around a gym for an hour to the point of collapse with 20 strangers, the TV wins outright, right? Even though you know deep down that not doing any exercise will eventually take its toll, it's just too much like hard work. However, exercise gives us more energy, reduces stress, makes us more capable and is highly addictive. And that's without listing any of the long-term health benefits. Overturning this 'hard work' excuse is what The Accumulator™ manages to do because it starts small and gradually builds as you begin to feel better in yourself and realise some of the benefits to be gained from regular exercise. Then, before you know it, you're working up a sweat, burning fat, changing your body and learning to love exercise.

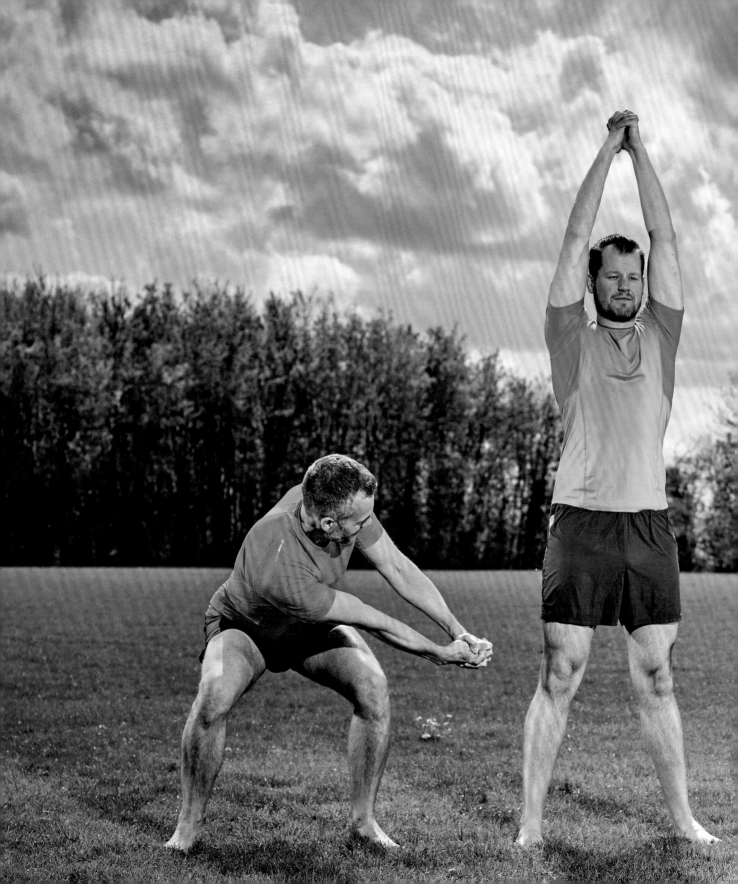

Accumulating exercises

THE ACCUMULATOR™ WORKOUT IS DESIGNED TO TEACH YOU HOW TO MOVE THE WAY YOUR BODY WANTS YOU TO, IT WILL HELP TO MAKE YOU FITTER IN EVERY ASPECT OF YOUR LIFE AND IT WILL CHALLENGE YOU TO WORK HARDER AS THE MONTH PROGRESSES. LET'S TURN THE PAGE AND GET STUCK IN. YOU CAN SEE VIDEO DEMONSTRATIONS OF EACH EXERCISE AT WWW.THEACCUMULATOR.NET.

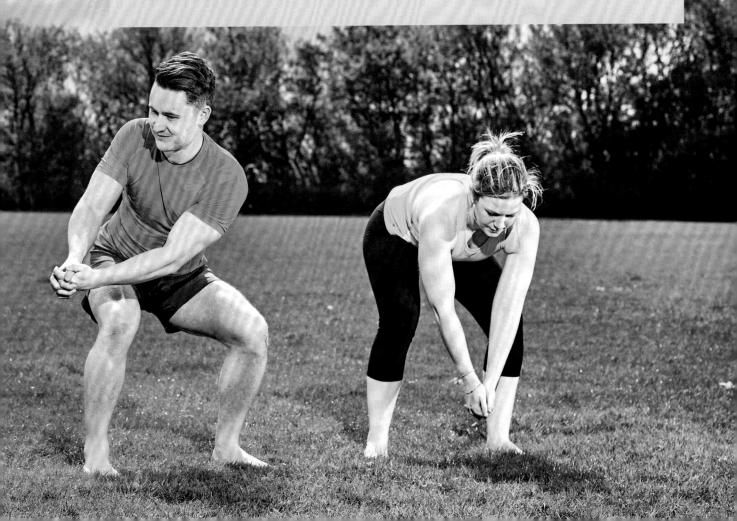

The Accumulator™ anatomy

I'S IMPORTANT FOR YOU TO KNOW WHICH MUSCLES YOU'LL BE USING FOR EACH EXERCISE BECAUSE IF YOU'RE NOT FEELING IT IN THE RIGHT PLACES, THERE'S A PRETTY BIG CHANCE THAT YOU'RE NOT DOING THE EXERCISE CORRECTLY. YOU'LL FIND A FULL LIST OF THE MAJOR MUSCLES USED IN EACH EXERCISE ON THE FOLLOWING PAGES. THIS PAGE WILL HELP YOU TO FIND THOSE MUSCLES ON YOUR OWN BODY SO YOU KNOW EXACTLY WHAT'S WORKING WHERE.

FROM THE FRONT

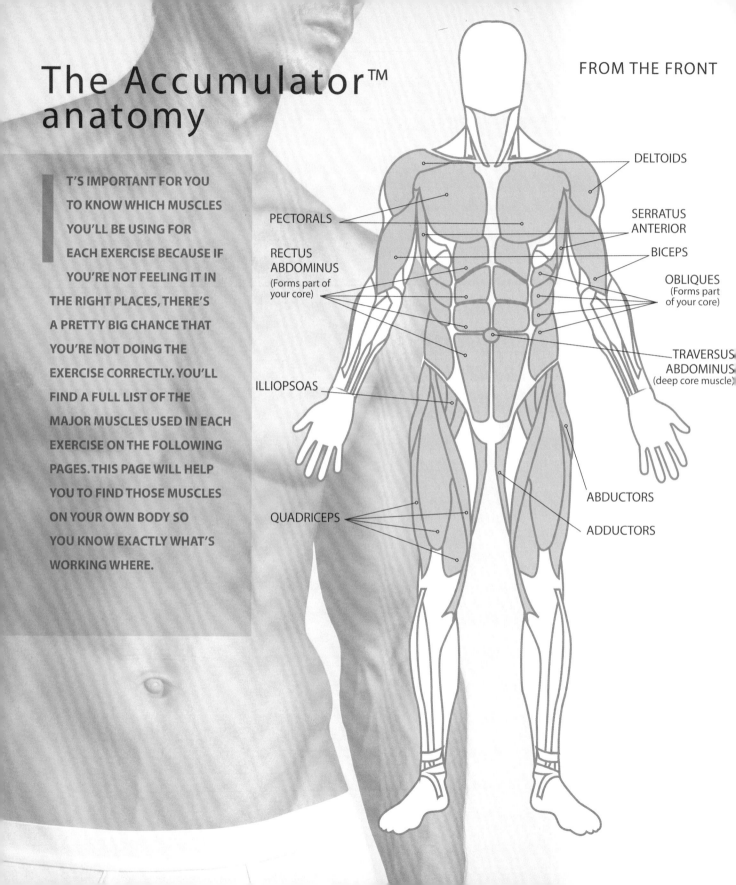

DELTOIDS

PECTORALS

SERRATUS ANTERIOR

RECTUS ABDOMINUS
(Forms part of your core)

BICEPS

OBLIQUES
(Forms part of your core)

TRAVERSUS ABDOMINUS
(deep core muscle)

ILLIOPSOAS

ABDUCTORS

QUADRICEPS

ADDUCTORS

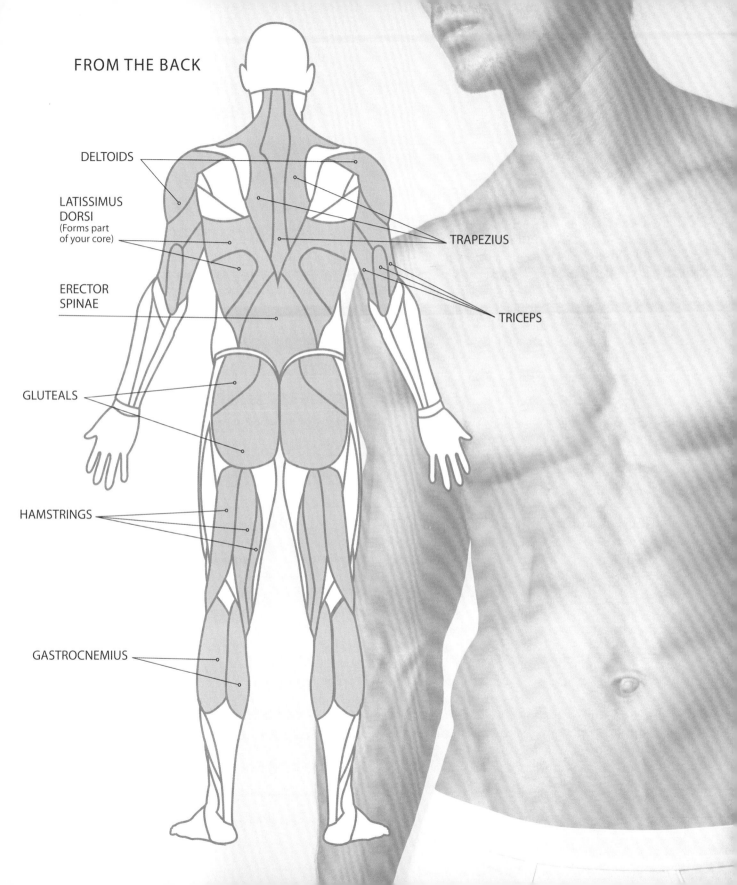

FROM THE BACK

DELTOIDS

LATISSIMUS
DORSI
(Forms part
of your core)

ERECTOR
SPINAE

GLUTEALS

HAMSTRINGS

GASTROCNEMIUS

TRAPEZIUS

TRICEPS

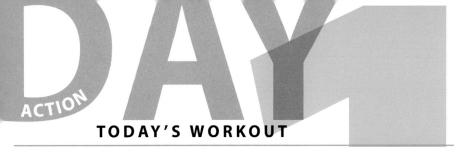

TODAY'S WORKOUT

PERFORM TODAY'S EXERCISE FOR 20 SECONDS, REST FOR 10 SECONDS AND REPEAT FOR 20 SECONDS.

SQUAT

squat

MUSCLES USED: Quadriceps/thighs, Gluteals/butt, Adductors/inside of thighs, Gastrocnemius/calves, Hamstrings, Illiopsoas/hip flexors, Core.

WHAT IT'S GOOD FOR? Perfecting squats will help you with sitting down and standing up, jumping and running, and forms the basis of many other everyday movements.

WHY SHOULD YOU DO IT? Whenever we sit down, we squat. When we jump, we start from a squat. A full squat with your butt close to the floor is actually your body's default sitting position. Before chairs were invented we would spend much of our time sitting in a full squat position. Even now in some cultures squatting is the norm for sitting, eating or going to the toilet. We all have the right equipment to squat all the way to the floor but many of us have simply lost this ability as we don't need to lower our butts below chair height. In fact, many people lack the strength to even sit in a chair in a controlled manner and instead resort to 'falling' into it or using the arm rests to support their weight as they lower themselves down.

The full squat is without question the best one you can do. It recruits more muscle fibres in your butt and thighs than a half squat, and demands a much higher level of flexibility, mobility and strength in many parts of your body – from your shoulders right down to your feet. Whereas sitting in a chair requires very little effort, the full squat utilises many of your muscles, especially ones in your core and lower back.

If you can't already perform a full squat, there could be several reasons why this is so. A weak core, tight lower back, immobility in the hips, weak gluteal muscles (in your butt) and even tightness in your calves and Achilles tendon can be contributory factors. However, with some stretching and practice it may be possible. There are two versions of the squat here, the second of which is a full one.

Version 1

- Stand with your feet facing forwards, slightly wider than hip-width apart. Your big toes should be roughly pointing in the same direction as each other.

- Extend your arms straight out in front of you as you squat.

- Bend at the knees and hips as if you are about to sit in a chair.

- When your butt is at the same height as your knees, push yourself back up by squeezing your butt.

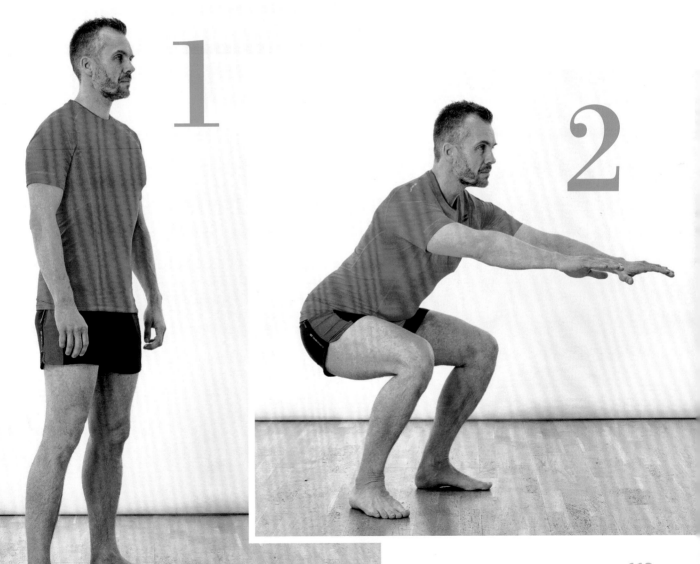

squat

Version 2

- Stand with your feet facing forwards, slightly wider than hip-width apart. Your big toes should be roughly pointing in the same direction.

- Extend your arms straight out in front of you as you squat.

- Bend at the knees and hips as if you are about to sit in a chair.

- Continue beyond knee height until the backs of your thighs touch your calves and your butt is close to the floor. Make sure your tailbone does not tuck underneath you.

- Return to the starting position by squeezing your butt. Try to avoid the temptation to bounce back up.

WHAT ELSE SHOULD I KNOW?

For both versions of the squat, make sure your feet remain flat on the floor. Be careful that you don't roll in or out at the ankles either. Your knees should always point forwards and should not get closer to each other as you get lower. Keep your weight on the balls of your feet and not on your heels. Your big toes should always remain in the same position too. Look ahead of you and not towards the floor.

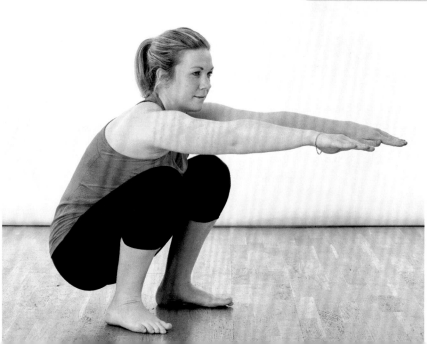

2DAY

ACTION

TODAY'S WORKOUT

PERFORM TODAY'S EXERCISE FOR 20 SECONDS, REST FOR 10 SECONDS AND REPEAT FOR 20 SECONDS. REST FOR 20 SECONDS BEFORE GOING BACK TO REPEAT YESTERDAY'S EXERCISE.

TWISTED SIDE LUNGE   SQUAT

twisted side lunge

MUSCLES USED: Quadriceps/thighs, Gluteals/butt, Adductors/inside of thighs, Gastrocnemius/calves, Hamstrings, Illiopsoas/hip flexors, Core (especially obliques), Latissimus dorsi/middle back.

WHAT IT'S GOOD FOR? Everyday movement, running, all sports (especially racquet sports).

WHY SHOULD YOU DO IT? This type of stepping and reaching movement is something you will find yourself doing in various forms on a daily basis. Lunging to one side fires up an important little muscle on the side of your butt that can become weak with under-use, but which is important for helping to stabilise your leg at the hip and prevent it from rotating inwards (think knocking knees). The primary job of the muscle group known as your core is to stabilise your spine. Our trunk rotates in many ways, hundreds of times each day. A strong core and back prevents this movement from causing back pain.

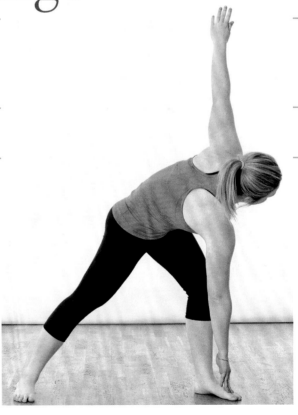

ACCUMULATOR ACTION **115**

2 twisted side lunge

Version 1

- Stand with your feet hip-width apart and arms down by your side.

- Take a large step to the left while bending at the hip and knee. Your right leg should remain straight.

- Turn your left foot slightly out as you land and keep both feet flat on the floor.

- At the same time, lean slightly forwards and turn to your left, reaching down to touch your left foot with your right hand.

- Return to the starting position and repeat in the other direction.

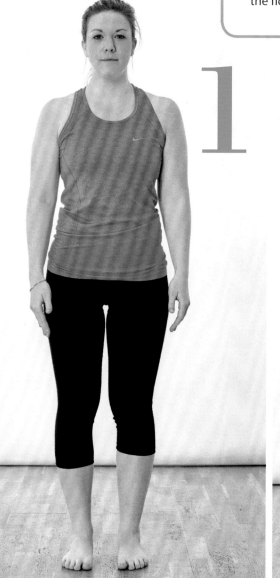

1

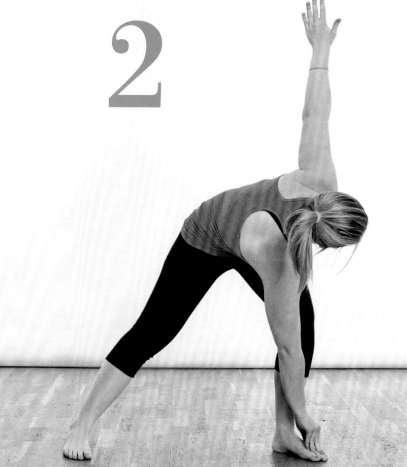

2

Version 2

- Stand with your feet hip-width apart and arms down by your side.

- Take a large step to the left while bending at the hip and knee. Your right leg should remain straight.

- Turn your left foot slightly out as you land and keep both feet flat on the floor.

- At the same time, lean slightly forwards and turn to your left, reaching down to touch your left foot with your right hand.

- Jump up back to the starting position and repeat with the other leg.

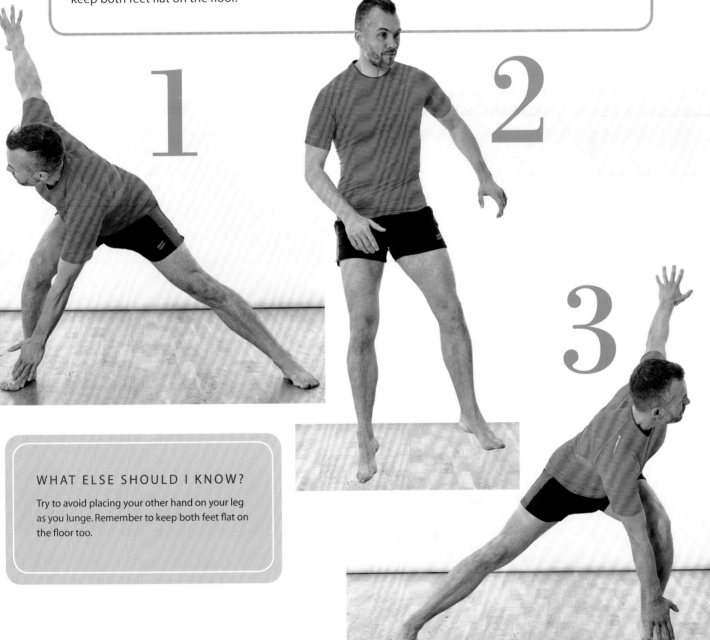

WHAT ELSE SHOULD I KNOW?

Try to avoid placing your other hand on your leg as you lunge. Remember to keep both feet flat on the floor too.

DAY 3

TODAY'S WORKOUT

PERFORM TODAY'S EXERCISE FOR 20 SECONDS, REST FOR 10 SECONDS AND REPEAT FOR 20 SECONDS. REST FOR 20 SECONDS BEFORE GOING BACK TO REPEAT YESTERDAY'S EXERCISE AND CONTINUE RIGHT BACK TO DAY 1.

PRESS-UP

TWISTED SIDE LUNGE

SQUAT

press-up

MUSCLES USED: Pectorals/chest, Triceps/back of arms, Deltoids/shoulders, Serratus anterior (under your armpits), Core.

WHAT IT'S GOOD FOR? Pushing, throwing, core strength, stability.

WHY SHOULD YOU DO IT? This is one exercise I think everyone should be able to do well. Not only will it help to improve your strength for anything that involves pushing or throwing, but it also enables many of the major muscles above your waistband to work as a team. One of the advantages of doing a press-up as opposed to a chest press with weights has to do with your core. A press-up works your chest and arms to push you away from the ground, but your core also has to do some work to keep your posture in perfect check. Lying on your back to do a chest press means your core doesn't need to do much at all. Besides, when do you have to push anything away from you while lying on your back in everyday life?

MAKE IT EASIER!

If you find this position too hard, try placing your hands on something that raises them higher than your knees (such as a step).

Version 1

- Get into position by lying face down on the floor with your feet hip-width apart.

- With your fingers spread, place your hands flat on the floor either side of your chest so they are underneath your elbows.

- Rotate your hands until your elbows point to around 4 o'clock and 8 o'clock.

- Push yourself up until your arms are straight.

Your knees should be on the floor and you should have a straight posture from the back of your knees to the top of your head.

- Lower yourself down by bending your elbows. Make sure you maintain your posture (don't arch your back).

- Try to lower yourself until your nose or chest touches the floor before pushing back to the starting position.

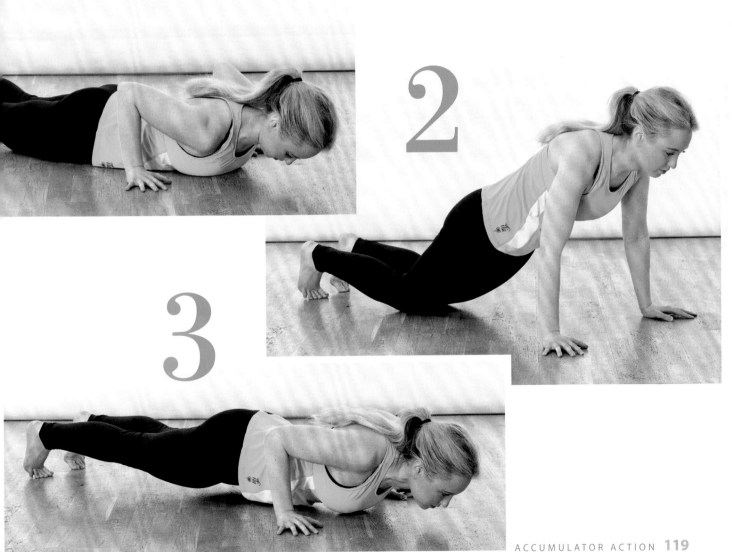

3 press up

Version 2

- Get into position by lying face down on the floor with your feet hip-width apart.

- With your fingers spread, place your hands flat on the floor either side of your chest so they are underneath your elbows.

- Rotate your hands until your elbows point to around 4 o'clock and 8 o'clock.

- Push yourself up until your arms are straight. Your toes should be on the floor and you should have a straight posture from the back of your heels to the top of your head.

- Lower yourself down by bending your elbows. Make sure you maintain your posture (don't arch your back).

- Try to lower yourself until your nose or chest touches the floor before pushing back to the starting position.

1

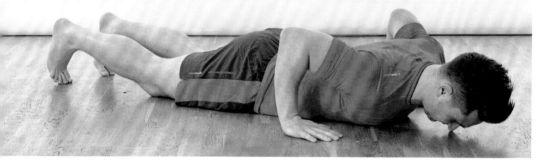

2

WHAT ELSE SHOULD I KNOW?

Posture is very important with a push-up. Make sure you don't look down towards your hips – you should be looking at the floor directly below you. Also be careful not to let your hips drop, your back arch or your butt to lift up in the air. At the top of the movement try to avoid locking your elbows; keep the joint soft. Watch you speed too. If you can do more than 10 repetitions in the 20 seconds you need to slow down.

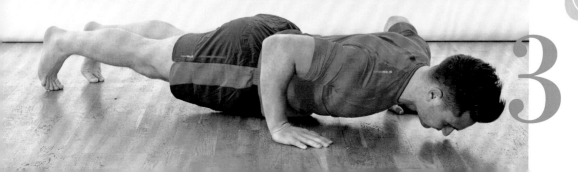

3

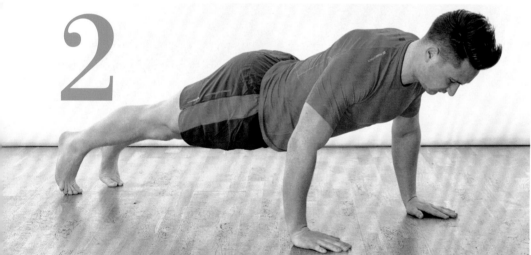

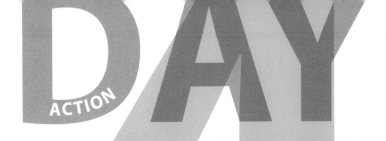

TODAY'S WORKOUT

PERFORM TODAY'S EXERCISE FOR 20 SECONDS, REST FOR 10 SECONDS AND REPEAT FOR 20 SECONDS. REST FOR 20 SECONDS BEFORE GOING BACK TO REPEAT YESTERDAY'S EXERCISE AND CONTINUE RIGHT BACK TO DAY 1.

DEAD LIFT

PRESS-UP

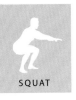
TWISTED SIDE LUNGE

SQUAT

dead lift

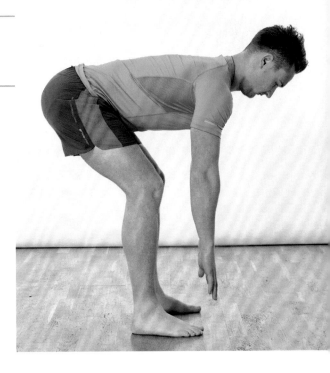

MUSCLES USED: Hamstrings/back of thighs, Gluteals/butt, Quadriceps/thighs, Latissimus dorsi/middle back, Core.

WHAT IT'S GOOD FOR? Picking up things from the floor, making the muscles and joints in your butt work properly, running, core strength, stability.

WHY SHOULD YOU DO IT? I've seen many variations of this exercise but this is the one I think works the best. However, it may take a few repetitions to get it right so you don't feel it in your lower back. If you spend much of your time sitting down, the muscles in your butt will be weak and therefore may be difficult to activate. With practice though, this exercise will help to switch on your butt muscles, make them stronger and protect your lower back.

Running with proper form activates the muscles at the back of your thighs and your butt as your leg lifts. The dead lift will not only make these muscles stronger, but it also teaches them to work as a team. And if you need any more reasons to do dead lifts, just think about all the times you need to pick up something from the floor.

4 deadlift

Version 1

- Stand with your feet shoulder-width apart.

- Bend at the hips until you are facing the floor. Keep your back straight and let your arms extend towards the floor.

- At the same time, push your butt out behind you, making sure you don't tip back on your feet. At this stage you should feel a pull in your hamstrings.

- Squeeze your butt as hard as you can to push yourself back to the starting position.

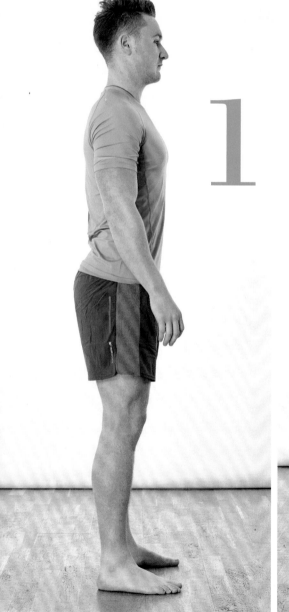

1

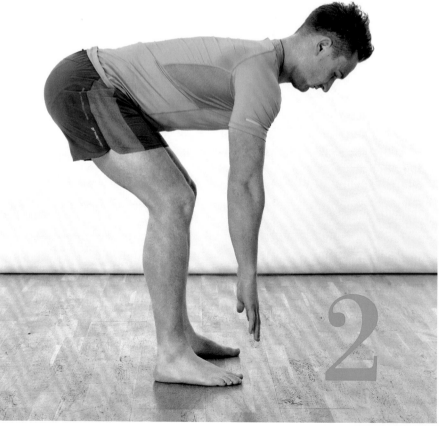

2

Version 2

- Stand on one leg (for this explanation, let's start with your left leg). Your arms should be by your side.

- Bend at the hip and send your other leg out behind you (this acts as a counterbalance). Keep your back straight.

- At the same time, reach down with your right hand to touch your left foot. The slight rotation will activate the muscles in your upper and middle back as well as your core.

- Squeeze your butt as hard as you can to push yourself back to the starting position.

- As this is a single-leg variation you can choose to do either one or two rounds of 20 seconds for each leg.

WHAT ELSE SHOULD I KNOW?

If you feel version 2 in your calves more than your hamstrings and butt, this could be because you are using your foot and ankle to balance too much, and your core not enough. Focus on contracting your core unit harder and your balance should improve. If you're still finding this hard, use a wall or stable object nearby to help you balance. Or continue with version 1 until your technique improves.

If you begin to feel this in your lower back, check your posture is correct by looking in a mirror, or ask someone to take a photo. Squeezing your butt will push you back upright and save the smaller muscles in your lower back from over-working.

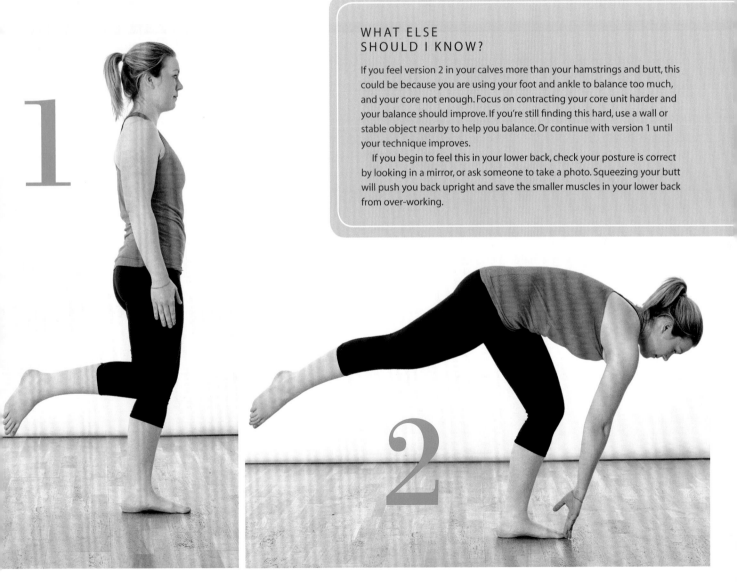

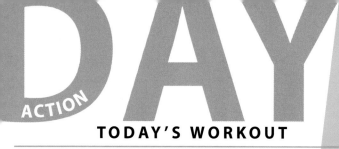

ACTION

DAY 5

TODAY'S WORKOUT

PERFORM TODAY'S EXERCISE FOR 20 SECONDS, REST FOR 10 SECONDS AND REPEAT FOR 20 SECONDS. REST FOR 20 SECONDS BEFORE GOING BACK TO REPEAT YESTERDAY'S EXERCISE AND CONTINUE RIGHT BACK TO DAY 1.

RUSSIAN TWIST

DEAD LIFT

PRESS-UP

TWISTED SIDE LUNGE

SQUAT

TIP
Always look straight ahead – don't turn your gaze to follow your hands. If you begin feeling this in your lower back or hips more than everywhere else, stop, take a rest and try again or re-check your posture.

russian twist

MUSCLES USED: Core (especially obliques), Latissimus dorsi/middle back, Gluteals/butt.

WHAT IT'S GOOD FOR? Any movement that involves twisting or reaching, running (especially off-road running).

WHY SHOULD YOU DO IT? In my opinion, the core is one of the most important but under-used muscle groups we have. Your core is the collective term for the team of muscles between your chest and your hips. They are designed to work together and are there to stabilise your spine. When you perform any movement that involves rotating or reaching to one side (for example, lifting a baby from a car seat and out of a car) the two pairs of muscles at our sides called obliques work a little harder to make sure you don't damage your spine. The same goes for running and walking, both of which involve a rotation of the spine that needs help from your obliques. These muscles have to work a little harder when you move on a less stable, softer surface, which explains why your core hurts when you run on the beach.

Version 1

- Sit on the floor with your knees bent and just your heels on the floor (not the whole of your feet).

- Lean backwards slightly, making sure your upper-body posture remains straight (don't curl your back).

- Straighten your arms in front of you and put your palms together.

- Move your arms from left to right, making sure one arm doesn't become longer than the other (you'll know what this means when you start doing it).

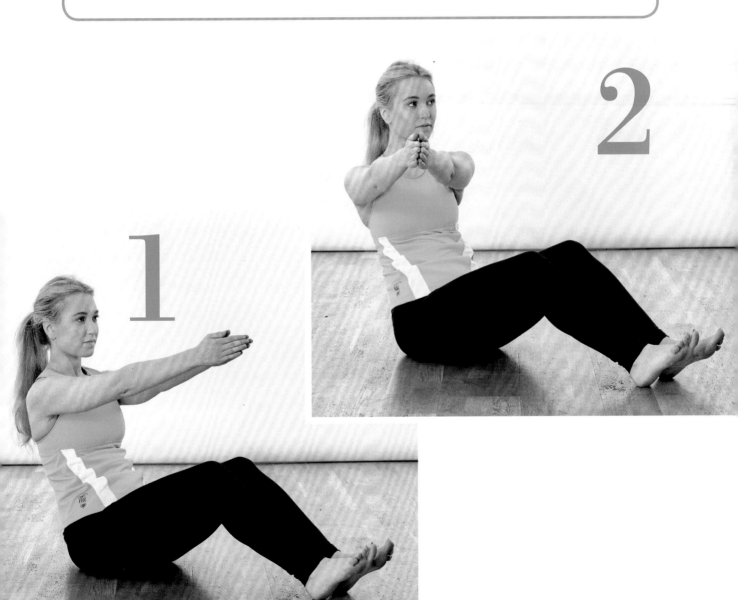

5 russian twist

Version 2

- Sit on the floor with your knees bent and your heels slightly off the floor.

- Lean backwards slightly, making sure your upper-body posture remains straight (don't curl your back).

- Straighten your arms in front of you and put your palms together.

- Move your arms from left to right, making sure one arm doesn't become longer than the other (you'll know what this means when you start doing it).

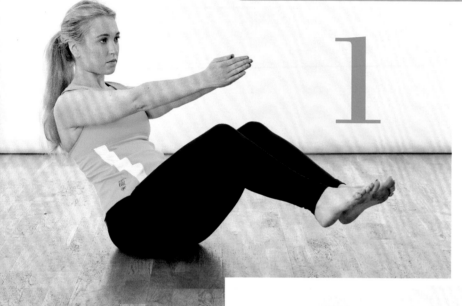

WHAT ELSE SHOULD I KNOW?

Version 2 is harder than it first appears because you will have to balance on your butt. Your posture becomes more important too, because if you are not balanced perfectly you'll notice either your lower back or the muscles in your legs working too much. Also be aware of how your legs are moving, or rather not moving. If your knees are shifting from side to side as you are, this is because your hips are rotating with you. Make smaller rotations until your hips remain still and work to build this up slowly.

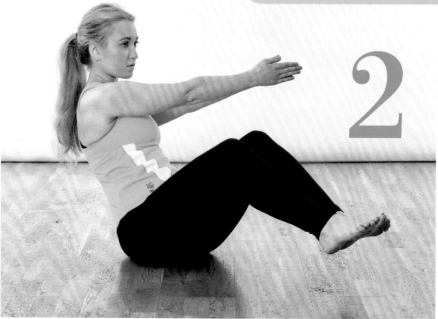

rest day

MUSCLES USED: None.

WHAT IT'S GOOD FOR? Recovery.

WHY SHOULD YOU DO IT? There are four rest days built into the workout plan and these are important for a number of reasons. If you're new to exercise, the last five days may have caused your body to feel a little sore (remember my earlier comments about DOMS)? However, it really doesn't have to all be about soreness. Rest days allow your body to recover and adapt to the new activities. Think of it as a day of growth. If you already exercise regularly, why not see this day off as an opportunity to do something different, such as going for a run or bike ride. Either way, trust me, you will be thankful for the rest days later in the month.

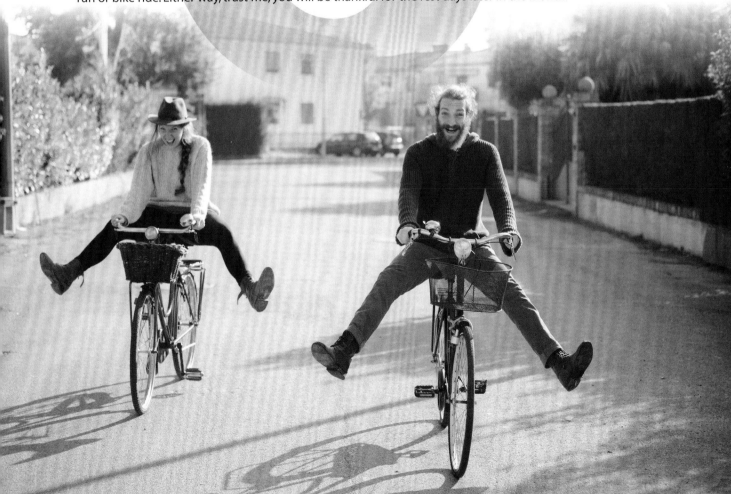

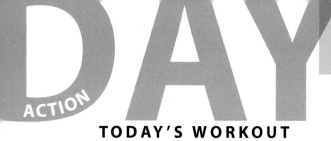

TODAY'S WORKOUT

PERFORM TODAY'S EXERCISE FOR 20 SECONDS, REST FOR 10 SECONDS AND REPEAT FOR 20 SECONDS. REST FOR 20 SECONDS BEFORE GOING BACK TO REPEAT YESTERDAY'S EXERCISE AND CONTINUE RIGHT BACK TO DAY 1.

  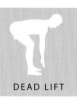

| BUTT RAISER | RUSSIAN TWIST | DEAD LIFT | PRESS-UP | TWISTED SIDE LUNGE | SQUAT |

butt raiser

MUSCLES USED: Gluteals/butt, Hamstrings/back of thighs, Core.

WHAT IT'S GOOD FOR? Jumping, running, climbing, lifting.

WHY SHOULD YOU DO IT? If you spend a lot of time sitting down your butt and core will both be weak and your hamstrings will be tight. This exercise will help to activate these muscles. In addition, having power in your behind gives you the edge when making a wide range of different movements. Oh and we all know a firm butt looks good, right?

HELP! I CAN'T FEEL THIS IN MY BUTT

If you feel this exercise in your shoulders or hamstrings more than your butt, you may need to practise activating your gluteal muscles before starting this exercise. It's quite common for the muscles in your butt to become lazy (especially if you sit down a lot). If this happens to you, try this quick exercise to activate your gluteals before doing today's exercise.

● Lie face down on the floor on your belly.

● Try to squeeze your buttocks together as hard as you can; imagine you're holding a pencil in between them and you're trying to stop someone from taking it away.

● If you get the contraction right your legs will lift away from the floor and rotate slightly outwards. Try 3 repetitions and hold each one for 5-10 seconds.

Version 1

- Sit on the floor with your legs in front of you.

- Draw one knee in until your foot is flat on the floor and level with the other knee. Place your hands on the floor behind you.

- Squeeze your butt and lift your hips as high as possible away from the floor.

- Keep the heel of your straight leg on the floor and move your hips directly upwards.

- Once you've reached the top, lower yourself back down (control this, don't drop) until your butt just touches the floor.

- Without taking a rest, head straight into the next repetition.

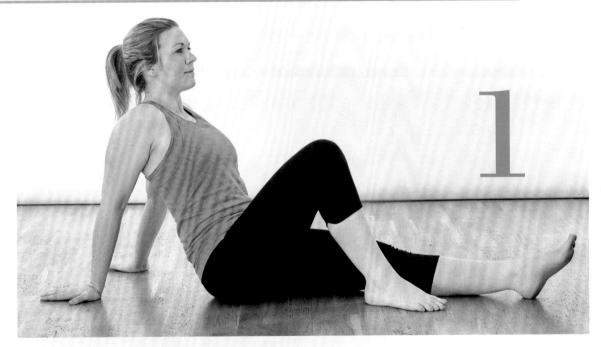

1

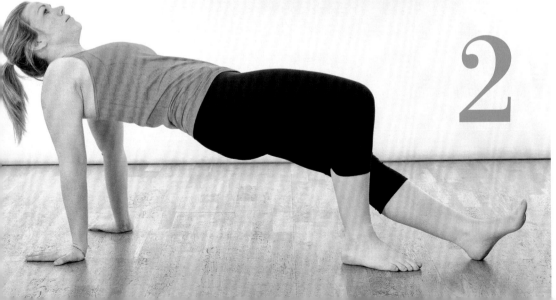

2

7 butt raiser

Version 2

- Sit on the floor with your legs in front of you.

- Draw one knee in until your foot is flat on the floor and level with the other knee. Place your hands on the floor behind you.

- Squeeze your butt and lift your hips as high as possible away from the floor.

- Raise your straight leg off the floor with you, making sure it goes no higher than your bent leg. Move your hips directly upwards.

- Once you've reached the top, hold the position for a second before lowering yourself back down (control this, don't drop) until your butt just touches the floor.

- Without taking a rest, head straight into the next repetition.

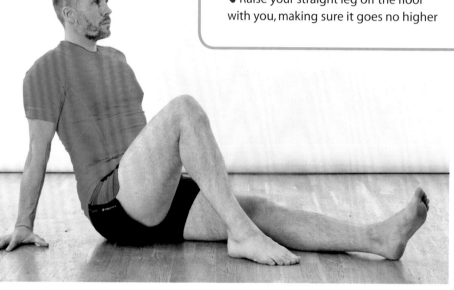

1

2

WHAT ELSE SHOULD I KNOW?

Try not to transfer your weight on to your arms and shoulders. Keep the foot of your bent leg flat on the floor. If your heel lifts at the top of the movement you need to move your foot further away from your hips. As these are both single leg exercises you can choose either one or two rounds of 20 seconds on each leg.

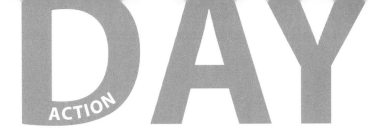
TODAY'S WORKOUT

PERFORM TODAY'S EXERCISE FOR 20 SECONDS, REST FOR 10 SECONDS AND REPEAT FOR 20 SECONDS. REST FOR 20 SECONDS BEFORE GOING BACK TO REPEAT YESTERDAY'S EXERCISE AND CONTINUE RIGHT BACK TO DAY 1.

   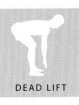   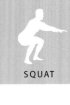

FORWARD LUNGE   BUTT RAISER   RUSSIAN TWIST   DEAD LIFT   PRESS-UP   TWISTED SIDE LUNGE   SQUAT

forward lunge
(prisoner lunge)

MUSCLES USED (VERSION 1): Gluteals/butt, Quadriceps/thighs, Hamstrings/ back of thighs, Gastrocnemius/calves, Core.

MUSCLES USED (VERSION 2): Gluteals/butt, Quadriceps/thighs, Hamstrings/ back of thighs, Gastrocnemius/calves, Core, Trapezius/upper back, Deltoids/ shoulders.

WHAT IT'S GOOD FOR? Throwing, jumping, striding, running, climbing, many sports.

WHY SHOULD YOU DO IT? Many people find the forward lunge is quite difficult to do properly. If you're new to exercise or haven't done lunges for some time, you may have weak or tight muscles, which can make this movement tricky to do correctly. Another major factor that enables correct lunging is good flexibility in your feet. Many of us have fairly weak feet and bending up on to our toes can be either painful or very difficult. If you run into problems bending your toes during the lunge (or any other exercise, for that matter) try some stretches that will help to mobilise your feet and toes.

Lunges are a fundamental movement and everyone should be able to do them with good form. If you play any racquet sport, they are a must since those games require you to use similar movements and doing this form of strength training can help prevent injury. Away from the court, you lunge to some degree while doing everyday activities such as vacuuming, sweeping or working in the garden, so being able to do it properly is an important skill to get right. A degree of balance is required and Version 2 makes balancing harder, further challenging your core, as well as working the muscles in your upper back and shoulders.

8 forward lunge (prisoner lunge)

Version 1

- Stand with your feet together and facing forwards.

- Take a big step forwards with your right leg and bend your knees until both legs are at a 90-degree angle.

- Your right foot should remain flat on the floor with your right knee directly above your right ankle.

- The toes of your left foot should be bent and your left knee should be directly underneath your left hip.

- Keep your upper body straight and look ahead (imagine your body is sandwiched between two panes of glass).

- Straighten your legs to return to the starting position and repeat the exercise by stepping forwards with your left leg.

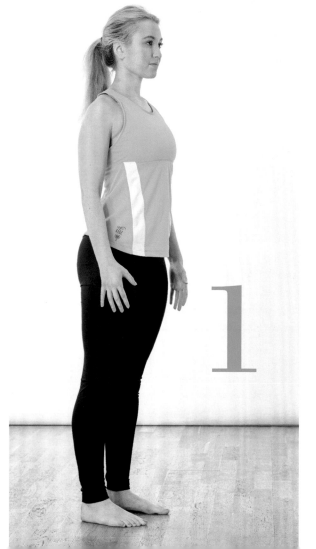

1

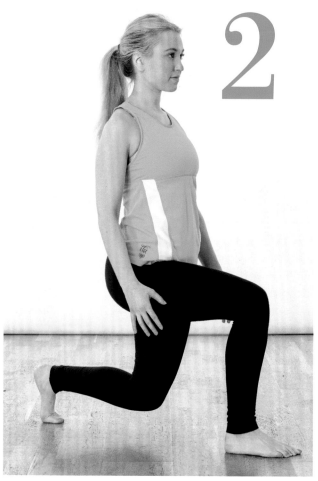

2

Version 2

- Stand with your feet together and facing forwards.

- Interlock your fingers and place your palms on the back of your head. Pull your elbows back until you can feel a squeeze in between your shoulder blades. Be careful not to push your head forwards. Keep your arms in this position throughout the exercise.

- Take a big step forwards with your right leg and bend your knees until both legs are at a 90-degree angle.

- Your right foot should remain flat on the floor with your right knee directly above your right ankle.

- The toes of your left foot should be bent and your left knee should be directly underneath your left hip.

- Keep your upper body straight and look ahead (imagine your body is sandwiched between two panes of glass).

- Straighten your legs to return to the starting position and repeat the exercise by stepping forwards with your left leg.

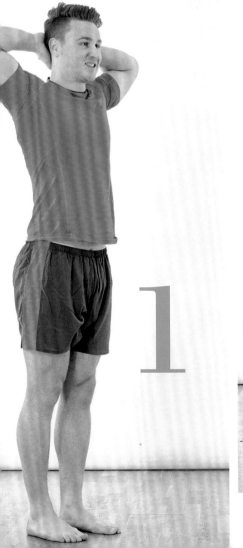

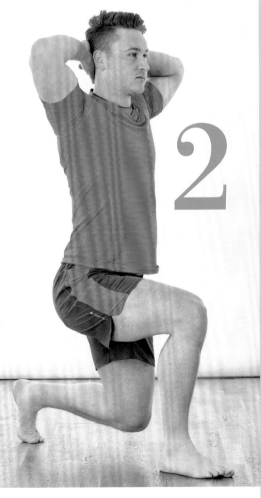

WHAT ELSE SHOULD I KNOW?

Remember to bend your toes at the back and make sure your heel is not rolling in or out. Also make sure your feet are not positioned wider apart than your hips and that your front knee does not bend inwards – it should remain in line with your hip. If you find this tricky there could be a number of reasons why. You have a little muscle on the outside of your butt that helps to keep your knee from rolling in during a lunge. If you find it hard to control your knee during this exercise, this muscle maybe the culprit. It's possible to re-activate this muscle but it can take some practice. Try this:

- Lie on your side facing the right. Your hips should be stacked directly on top of each other.

- Bend your left knee and extend your right leg straight out so your foot is slightly behind your hip.

- Hold this position for 30 seconds to 1 minute and you will feel the muscle on the outside of your butt activate to hold your leg in position.

- Repeat on the other side.

TODAY'S WORKOUT

PERFORM TODAY'S EXERCISE FOR 20 SECONDS, REST FOR 10 SECONDS AND REPEAT FOR 20 SECONDS. REST FOR 20 SECONDS BEFORE GOING BACK TO REPEAT YESTERDAY'S EXERCISE AND CONTINUE RIGHT BACK TO DAY 1.

| TOWEL ROW | FORWARD LUNGE | BUTT RAISER | RUSSIAN TWIST | DEAD LIFT | PRESS-UP | TWISTED SIDE LUNGE | SQUAT |

towel row

MUSCLES USED: Latissimus dorsi/middle back, Trapezius/upper back, Deltoids/shoulders, Biceps/upper arm.

WHAT IT'S GOOD FOR? Pulling, climbing, lifting, posture.

WHY SHOULD YOU DO IT? Bad posture can lead to many problems. If you have a job that involves sitting at a desk or driving, you will spend the vast majority of your time with your arms in front of your body. This can create tightness across your chest and conversely a weakness across your middle and upper back, which can result in a rounded posture called 'upper crossed syndrome' as your shoulders roll forwards. As a consequence of this imbalance it can become difficult to reach up above your head without arching your back. In order to establish whether you have this syndrome, lie on the floor on your back with your legs flat on the floor and your arms by your side. Now rotate your arms above your head and allow them to fall towards the floor behind your head without bending them. If your back arches or your arms simply fail to reach the floor, this could be indicative of 'upper crossed syndrome'. This exercise helps to strengthen these important postural muscles.

There is only 1 version today

- Take a small towel and roll it up lengthways.

- Lie face down on the floor with the towel at arm's length in front of you.

- With your arms straight, hold the towel at either end and pull it tight so it doesn't sag in the middle.

- Lift your arms away from the floor and bend them, drawing the towel in until it ends up underneath your chin.

- Straighten your arms again and keep them (and the towel) off the floor as you start again.

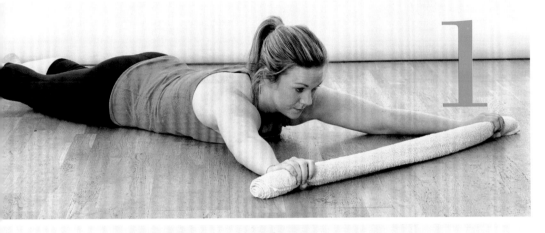

1

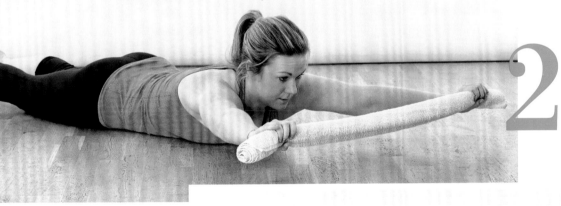

2

3

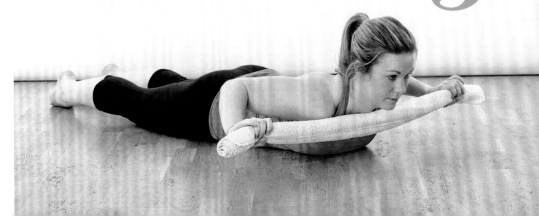

WHAT ELSE SHOULD I KNOW?

You should be able to do this without arching your back. If your back does arch, squeeze your shoulder blades tightly and lift your elbows higher as the towel comes towards you.

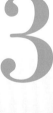

TODAY'S WORKOUT

PERFORM TODAY'S EXERCISE FOR 20 SECONDS, REST FOR 10 SECONDS AND REPEAT FOR 20 SECONDS. REST FOR 20 SECONDS BEFORE GOING BACK TO REPEAT YESTERDAY'S EXERCISE AND CONTINUE RIGHT BACK TO DAY 1.

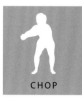 CHOP

 TOWEL ROW

 FORWARD LUNGE

 BUTT RAISER

 RUSSIAN TWIST

 DEAD LIFT

 PRESS-UP

 TWISTED SIDE LUNGE

 SQUAT

chop

MUSCLES USED (VERSION 1): Quadriceps/thighs, Gluteals/butt, Adductors/inside of thighs, Gastrocnemius/calves, Hamstrings, Illiopsoas/hip flexors, Latissimus dorsi/middle back, Core (especially obliques).

MUSCLES USED (VERSION 2) Quadriceps/thighs, Gluteals/butt Adductors/inside of thighs, Gastrocnemius/calves, Hamstrings, Illiopsoas/hip flexors, Latissimus dorsi/middle back, Deltoids/shoulders, Trapezius/upper back, Core (especially obliques).

WHAT IT'S GOOD FOR? Sitting down, jumping, running, throwing, rowing.

WHY SHOULD YOU DO IT? This is the first time we've put two exercises together, which will begin to take your breath away. The chopping movement you make with your arms has so many practical applications that it would be impossible to list them all here. In addition, the exercise targets all those muscles in your core that help with rotation.

Version 1

- Stand with your feet facing forwards, slightly wider than hip-width apart. Your big toes should be pointing in roughly the same direction as each other.

- Extend your arms straight out in front of you and in line with your shoulders. Clasp your hands together.

- Bend at the knees and hips as if you are about to sit in a chair.

- As you squat, rotate to the left and send your arms to the left. Your right shoulder should move closer to your left knee.

- At the same time drop your straight arms so they are close to your left hip.

- When your butt is at the same height as your knees, push yourself back up (by squeezing your butt) and return your arms to the starting position.

- Repeat, this time sending your arms to the right.

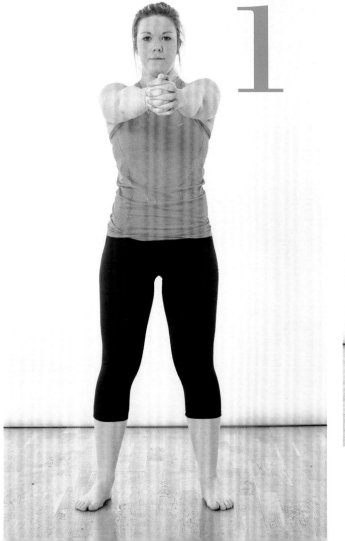

1

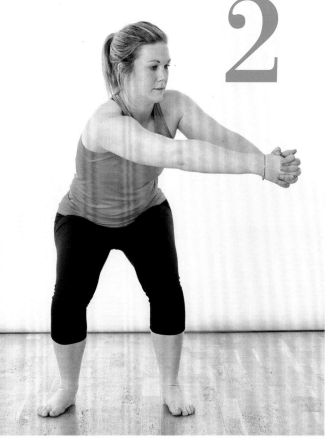

2

chop

10

Version 2

● Stand with your feet facing forwards, slightly wider than hip-width apart. Your big toes should be pointing in roughly the same direction as each other.

● Extend your arms straight above your head. Clasp your hands together.

● Bend at the knees and hips as if you are about to sit in a chair.

● As you squat, rotate to the left and send your arms to the left. Your right

shoulder should move closer to your left knee.

● At the same time drop your straight arms so they are close to your left hip.

● When your butt is at the same height as your knees, push yourself back up (by squeezing your butt) and return your arms to the starting position.

1

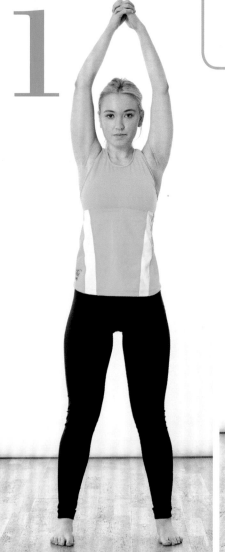

2

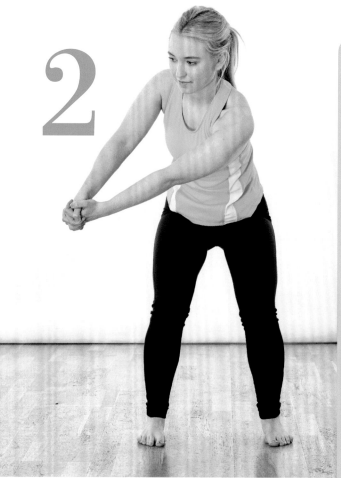

WHAT ELSE SHOULD I KNOW?

Try not to allow your arms to relax at all and avoid letting them swing from side to side. You should be in control of your arms at all times; they should remain straight and if you are rotating properly through your torso they will remain the same length as each other. If you begin to feel this exercise in your lower back, you may be tipping too far forwards when you squat. Be aware of your squatting technique and push through your butt rather than your lower back.

TODAY'S WORKOUT

PERFORM TODAY'S EXERCISE FOR 20 SECONDS, REST FOR 10 SECONDS AND REPEAT FOR 20 SECONDS. REST FOR 20 SECONDS BEFORE GOING BACK TO REPEAT YESTERDAY'S EXERCISE AND CONTINUE RIGHT BACK TO DAY 1.

 BOX JUMP
 CHOP
 TOWEL ROW
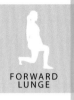 FORWARD LUNGE
 BUTT RAISER
 RUSSIAN TWIST
 DEAD LIFT
 PRESS-UP
 TWISTED SIDE LUNGE
 SQUAT

box jump

MUSCLES USED: Quadriceps/thighs, Gluteals/butt, Adductors/inside of thighs, Abductors/outside of thighs, Gastrocnemius/calves, Hamstrings, Illiopsoas/hip flexors.

WHAT IT'S GOOD FOR? Sitting down, jumping, running, all sports (especially racquet sports), coordination.

WHY SHOULD YOU DO IT? This is a great exercise to target the many tiny muscles around your hip joints as it involves moving your legs in different directions. It also works on that important butt muscle we were talking about on Day 7. Coordination and rhythm are skills many of us lose if we don't use them regularly and you'll find this fairly aerobic too.

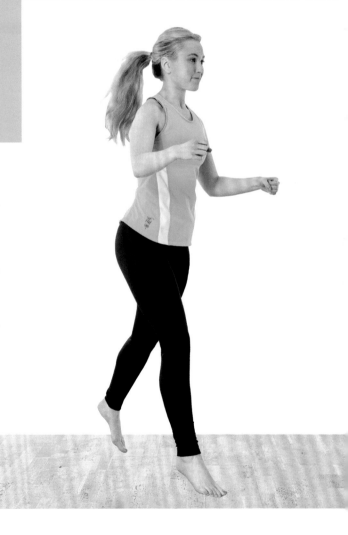

11 box jump

There is only 1 version today

- Imagine there's a square drawn on the floor and you are standing in the middle of it. Its corners are pointing away from you at roughly 2 o'clock, 5 o'clock, 8 o'clock and 11 o'clock.
- Jump so one foot lands on each opposite corner of your square (2 o'clock and 8 o'clock)
- Return to the middle and then jump to the other two corners (5 o'clock and 11 o'clock).

1

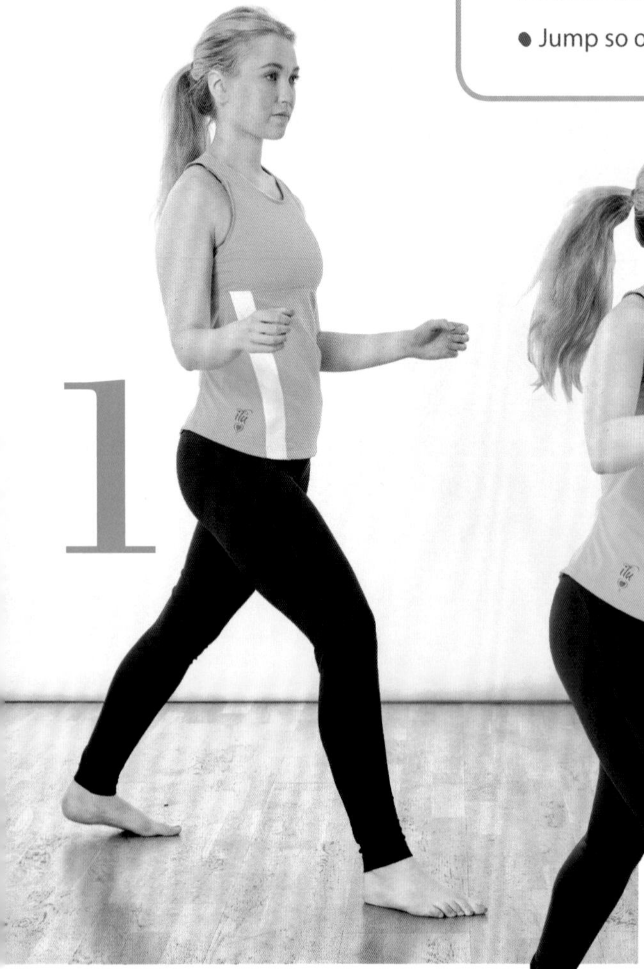

2

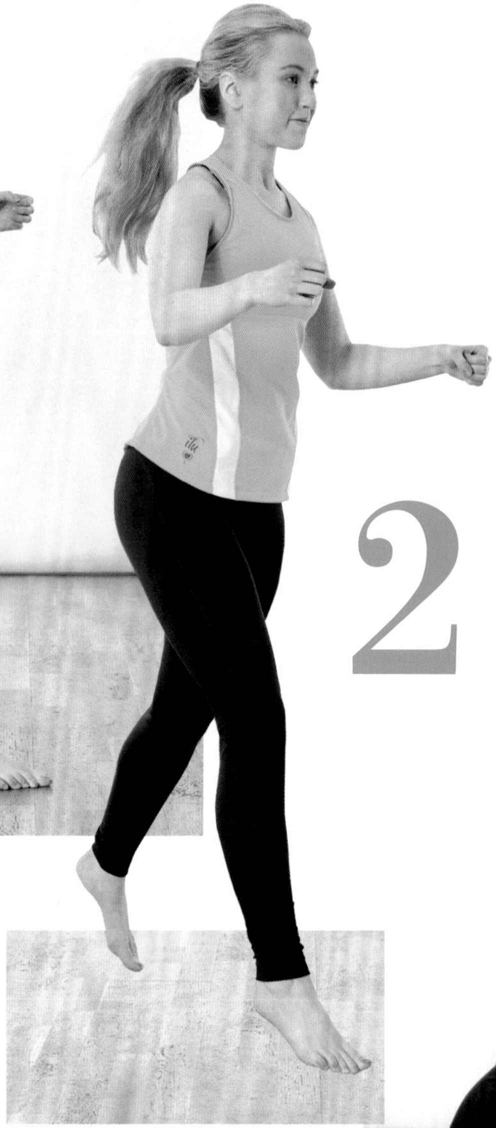

3

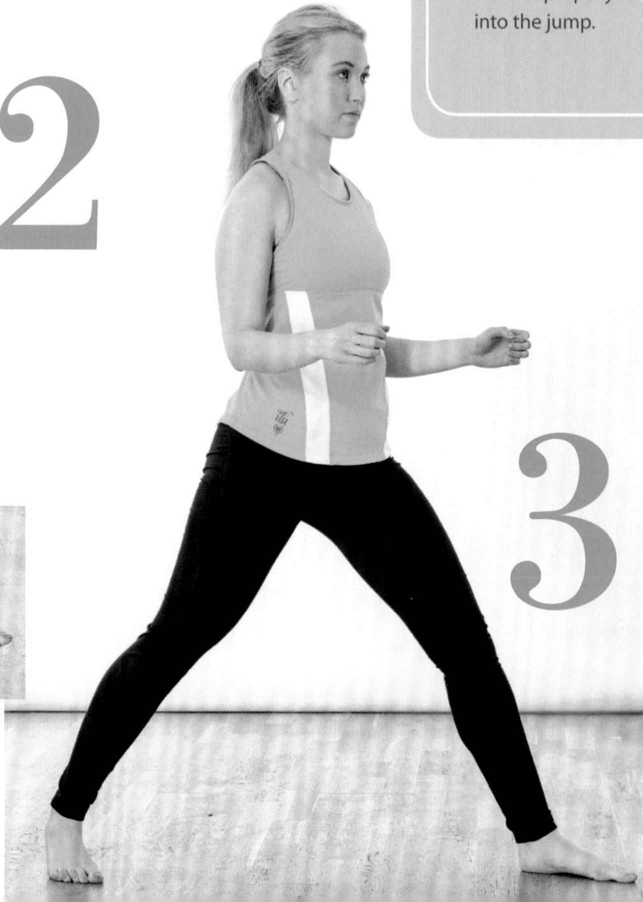

WHAT ELSE SHOULD I KNOW?

Even though you are sending your legs to diagonal corners of the box, your body should remain facing forwards. Bend your knees and use your arms to propel you into the jump.

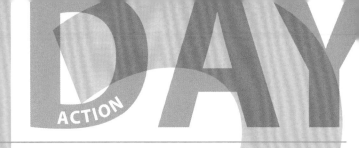

rest day

MUSCLES USED: None.

WHAT IT'S GOOD FOR? Recovery.

WHY SHOULD YOU DO IT? By now the rest day will start to become a welcome break. Remember, you can always take this rest on another day during the week if your muscles are sore then. Do make sure you don't skip your rest day altogether.

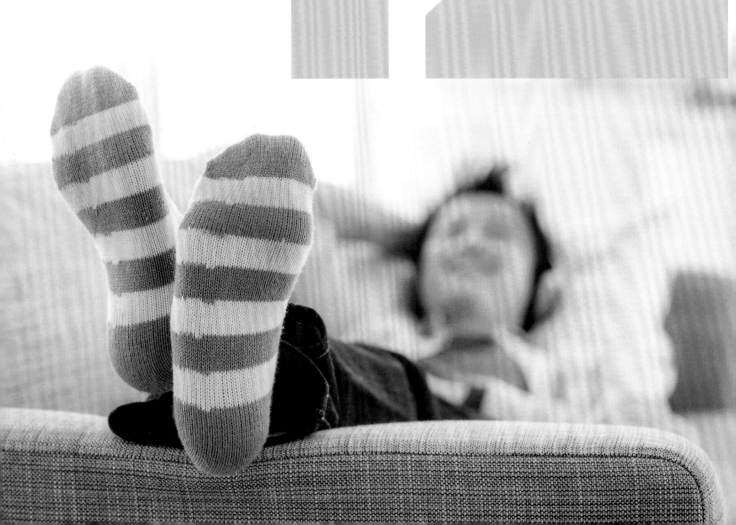

TODAY'S WORKOUT

PERFORM TODAY'S EXERCISE FOR 20 SECONDS, REST FOR 10 SECONDS AND REPEAT FOR 20 SECONDS. REST FOR 20 SECONDS BEFORE GOING BACK TO REPEAT YESTERDAY'S EXERCISE AND CONTINUE RIGHT BACK TO DAY 1.

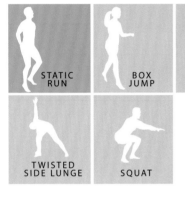

STATIC RUN | BOX JUMP | CHOP | TOWEL ROW | FORWARD LUNGE | BUTT RAISER | RUSSIAN TWIST | DEAD LIFT | PRESS-UP

TWISTED SIDE LUNGE | SQUAT

static run

MUSCLES USED: Quadriceps/thighs, Gluteals/butt, Adductors/inside of thighs, Abductors/outside of thighs, Gastrocnemius/calves, Hamstrings, Illiopsoas/hip flexors.

WHAT IT'S GOOD FOR? Jumping, running, all sports, aerobic capacity.

WHY SHOULD YOU DO IT? This simple cardiovascular exercise will get your heart racing. By the very nature of the workout every exercise is aerobic, but this one is especially vigorous. Obviously it's great for running, which is useful for many reasons and is something we should all be able to do.

- Run on the spot, making sure your heels touch the floor each time you land. You should naturally land on the balls of your feet.

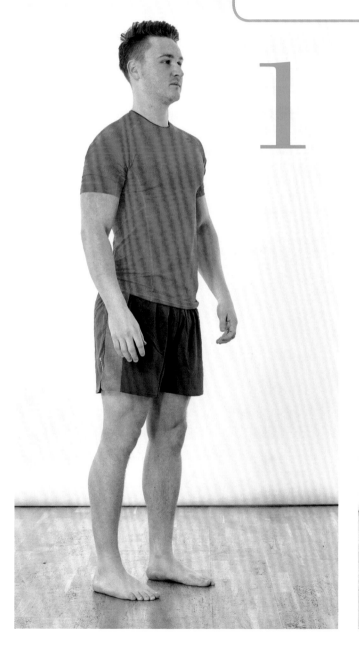

1

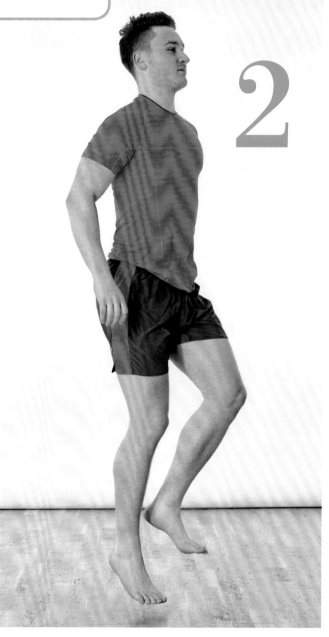

2

13 box jump

Version 2

- Run on the spot, making sure your heels touch the floor each time you land. You should naturally land on the balls of your feet.

- Hold your arms out in front of you with your arms bent and your elbows by your side. Turn your hands to face the floor and bring them closer together so they are in line with your knees.

- As you move, lift your knees high, until they touch your hands.

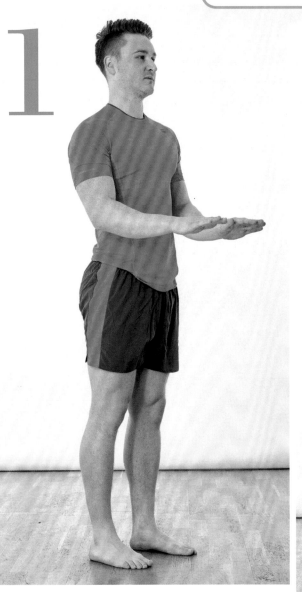

1

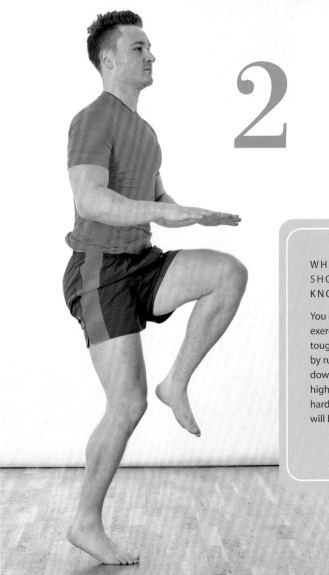

2

WHAT ELSE SHOULD I KNOW?

You could make this exercise an even tougher challenge by running up and down a step. The higher the step, the harder the action will be.

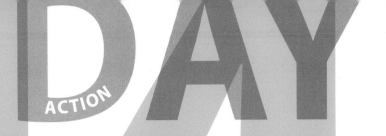
TODAY'S WORKOUT

PERFORM TODAY'S EXERCISE FOR 20 SECONDS, REST FOR 10 SECONDS AND REPEAT FOR 20 SECONDS. REST FOR 20 SECONDS BEFORE GOING BACK TO REPEAT YESTERDAY'S EXERCISE AND CONTINUE RIGHT BACK TO DAY 1.

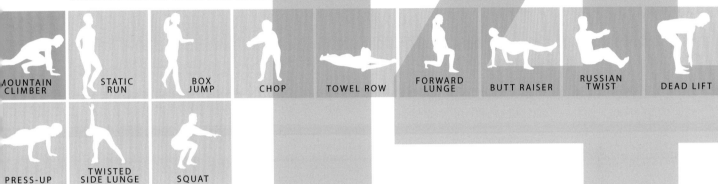

MOUNTAIN CLIMBER · STATIC RUN · BOX JUMP · CHOP · TOWEL ROW · FORWARD LUNGE · BUTT RAISER · RUSSIAN TWIST · DEAD LIFT · PRESS-UP · TWISTED SIDE LUNGE · SQUAT

Mountain climber

MUSCLES USED: Quadriceps/thighs, Gluteals/butt, Adductors/inside of thighs, Abductors/outside of thighs, Gastrocnemius/calves, Hamstrings, Illiopsoas/hip flexors, Deltoids/shoulders, Triceps, Core.

WHAT IT'S GOOD FOR? Jumping, running, crawling, climbing, all sports, aerobic capacity.

WHY SHOULD YOU DO IT? Climbing is one of our key primal movements, and even though our ape-like ancestors were equipped to climb better than we ever can, we have the potential to still be pretty good at it. Transferring the climbing movement pattern to the floor (facing the floor in a prone position) recruits your core, upper body, back and arms in much the same way as a plank or push-up. In fact, there's not much of your body that doesn't have to work when you perform this exercise.

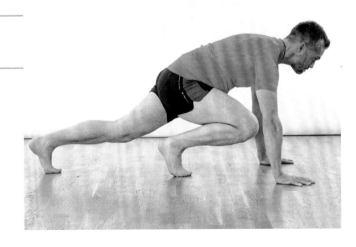

14 mountain climber

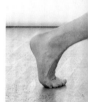

Version 1

- Start with your body facing the floor. Your arms should be straight and your hands on the floor directly underneath your shoulders. Your body should be straight with your feet behind you, hip-width apart and with your toes curled under.

- While maintaining this position, bend one leg and draw it in until your knee reaches your arm on the same side.

- Step back and repeat using the other leg.

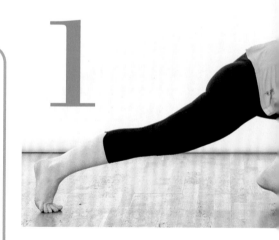

Version 2

- Start with your body facing the floor. Your arms should be straight and your hands should be on the floor directly underneath your shoulders. Your body should be straight with your feet behind you, hip-width apart and with your toes curled under.

- While maintaining this position, push both feet away from the floor and jump one leg in until your knee reaches your arm on the same side.

- Jump back, and at the same time swap legs so as you land the other knee is bent and the first leg is straight.

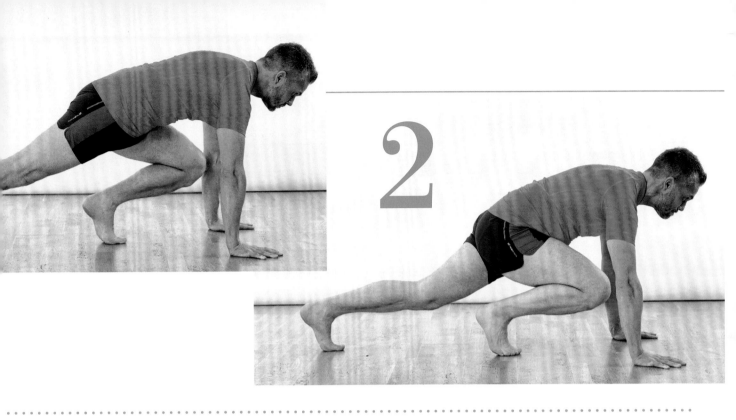

2

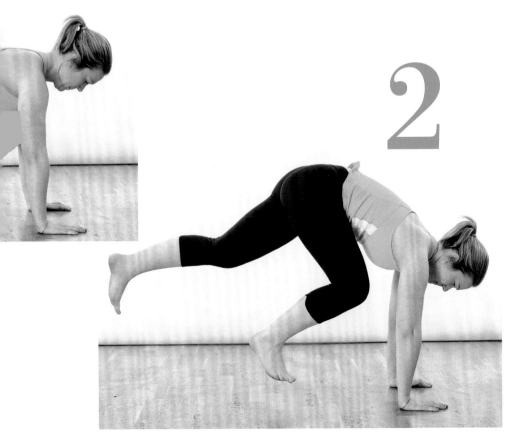

2

WHAT ELSE SHOULD I KNOW?

Squeezing your core muscles and butt will prevent your lower back from sagging (as in a push-up or plank). Be careful not to move your upper body backwards or tuck your pelvis underneath you so your knee and arm can touch. Your hands should be directly under your shoulders and your posture needs to be straight. Version 2 works much more aerobically than Version 1 by adding in the jumping, which makes the muscles in your legs and butt work that little bit harder. Remember to maintain your posture and keep in control of your movements.

TODAY'S WORKOUT

PERFORM TODAY'S EXERCISE FOR 20 SECONDS, REST FOR 10 SECONDS AND REPEAT FOR 20 SECONDS. REST FOR 20 SECONDS BEFORE GOING BACK TO REPEAT YESTERDAY'S EXERCISE AND CONTINUE RIGHT BACK TO DAY 1.

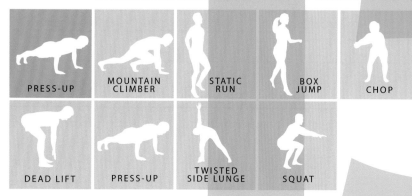

| PRESS-UP | MOUNTAIN CLIMBER | STATIC RUN | BOX JUMP | CHOP | TOWEL ROW | FORWARD LUNGE | BUTT RAISER | RUSSIAN TWIST |

| DEAD LIFT | PRESS-UP | TWISTED SIDE LUNGE | SQUAT |

press-up (reverse press-up)

REPEAT EXERCISE – SEE PAGE 116 FOR FULL DETAILS

You've now been doing press ups since Day 3 so they should be familiar by now. If you need to make them more challenging try a reverse press up instead. Start as you did for version 2, this time go towards the floor until your whole body makes contact with the ground at the same time. Allow your arms to relax slightly before pushing back up so your whole body should leave the floor at exactly the same time. Check out the video for this at www.theaccumulator.net.

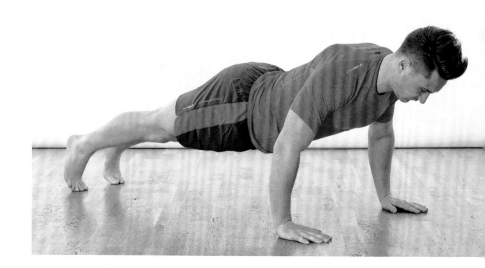

TODAY'S WORKOUT

PERFORM TODAY'S EXERCISE FOR 20 SECONDS, REST FOR 10 SECONDS AND REPEAT FOR 20 SECONDS. REST FOR 20 SECONDS BEFORE GOING BACK TO REPEAT YESTERDAY'S EXERCISE AND CONTINUE RIGHT BACK TO DAY 1.

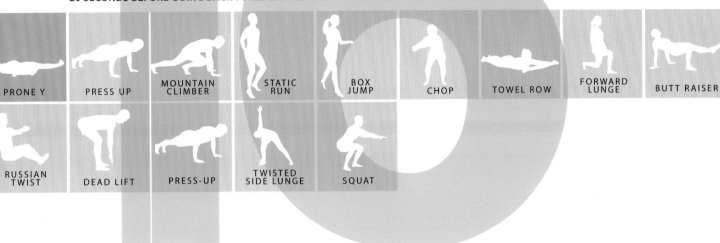

| PRONE Y | PRESS UP | MOUNTAIN CLIMBER | STATIC RUN | BOX JUMP | CHOP | TOWEL ROW | FORWARD LUNGE | BUTT RAISER |

| RUSSIAN TWIST | DEAD LIFT | PRESS-UP | TWISTED SIDE LUNGE | SQUAT |

prone Y

MUSCLES USED: Trapezius/upper back, Deltoids/shoulders, Latissimus dorsi/middle back.

WHAT IT'S GOOD FOR? Improving upper-body posture, throwing, flexibility, posture, pulling, lifting.

WHY SHOULD YOU DO IT? The Prone Y is a very small but very tough exercise that focuses on a much smaller percentage of your body than many other exercises in The Accumulator™. There's a good reason for this: this set of muscles can be much under-used in modern life and grow very weak, therefore they require some specific work in isolation. Like the towel row, this exercise also addresses any muscular imbalances in your upper body and improves your posture.

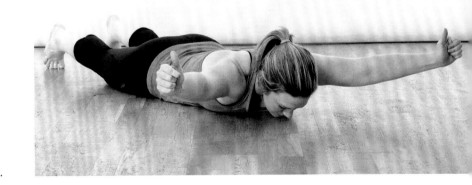

prone Y

Version 1

- Lie face down on the floor.

- Take your arms straight out in front of your head so your body makes a Y shape.

- Turn your hands around, make a fist and point your thumbs towards the ceiling.

- Keeping your chin on the floor, lift both arms straight in the air while maintaining that Y shape.

- Lift your arms as high as you can and slowly return to the floor before repeating the movement.

Version 2

- Lie face down on the floor with your feet together.

- Take your arms straight out in front of your head so your body makes a Y shape.

- Turn your hands around, make a fist and point your thumbs towards the ceiling.

- Keeping your chin on the floor, lift both arms straight in the air while maintaining that Y shape.

- Lift your arms as high as you can.

- Slowly lower your arms until they hover just above the floor then return them to the higher position.

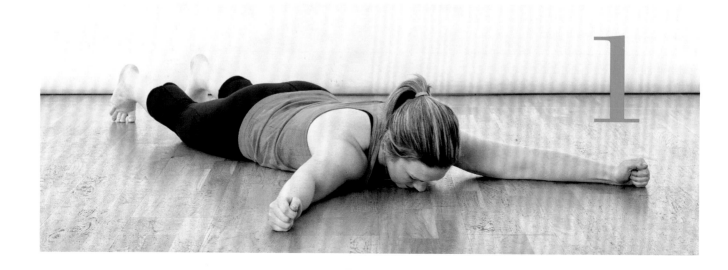

1

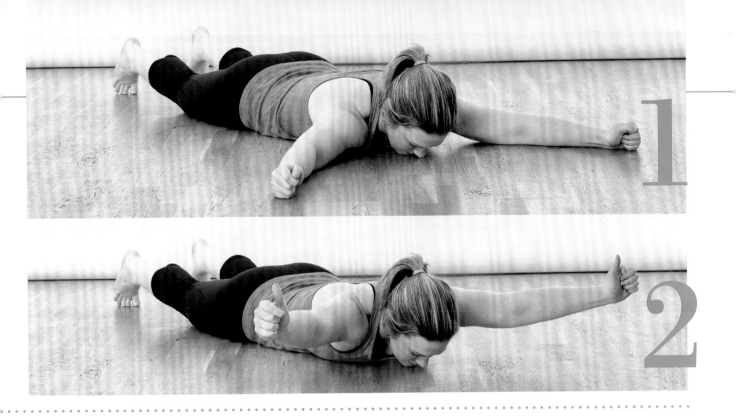

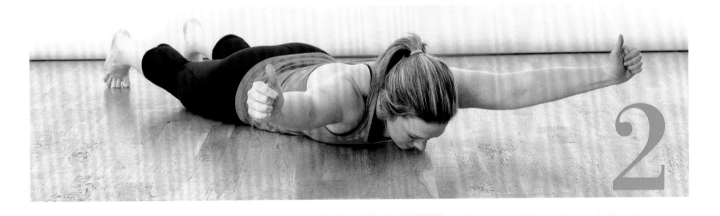

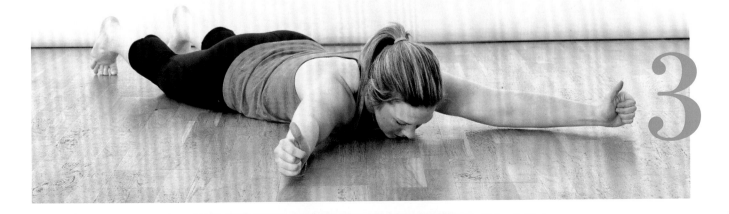

prone Y

Version 3

- Lie face down on the floor with your feet together.

- Take your arms straight out in front of your head so your body makes a Y shape.

- Turn your hands around, make a fist and point your thumbs towards the ceiling.

- Keeping your chin on the floor, lift both arms straight in the air while maintaining that Y shape.

- Lift your arms as high as you can.

- Maintain this position for the whole 20 seconds. Don't move.

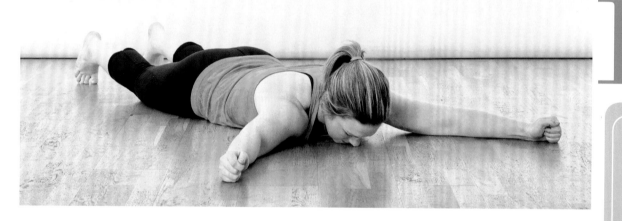

1

2

WHAT ELSE SHOULD I KNOW?

Don't be deceived by Version 3. This is actually much harder than it seems, so make sure you are capable of doing both Versions 1 and 2 before tackling it. Remember to keep your chin on the floor throughout as this will stop your back from arching and will help to activate the muscles in your upper back between your shoulder blades.

TODAY'S WORKOUT

PERFORM TODAY'S EXERCISE FOR 20 SECONDS, REST FOR 10 SECONDS AND REPEAT FOR 20 SECONDS. REST FOR 20 SECONDS BEFORE GOING BACK TO REPEAT YESTERDAY'S EXERCISE AND CONTINUE RIGHT BACK TO DAY 1.

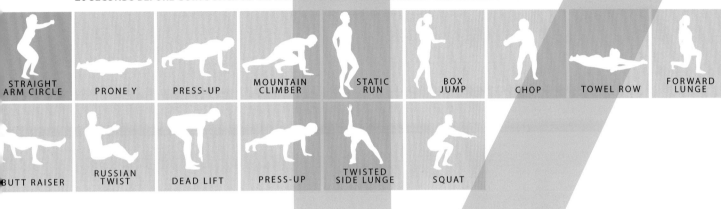

STRAIGHT ARM CIRCLE · PRONE Y · PRESS-UP · MOUNTAIN CLIMBER · STATIC RUN · BOX JUMP · CHOP · TOWEL ROW · FORWARD LUNGE

BUTT RAISER · RUSSIAN TWIST · DEAD LIFT · PRESS-UP · TWISTED SIDE LUNGE · SQUAT

straight arm circle

MUSCLES USED (VERSION 1): Trapezius/upper back, Deltoids/shoulders, Latissimus dorsi/middle back, core, Obliques/side of core.

MUSCLES USED (VERSION 2): Trapezius/upper back, Deltoids/shoulders, Latissimus dorsi/middle back, core, Obliques/side of core, Quads/thighs, Gluteals/butt, Hamstrings, Calves.

WHAT IT'S GOOD FOR? Improving upper-body posture, throwing, flexibility, running, climbing, racquet sports, pulling, lifting.

WHY SHOULD YOU DO IT? Today we're building on all the benefits from yesterday's exercise. This teaches you how to move fluidly through your core and incorporates all the muscles across your back as well as helping you extend your reach above your head. There's an awful lot going on here and getting this right is much harder than it may seem. Make sure you're confident that you've got Version 1 right before moving on. Version 2 essentially puts two exercises together by incorporating a squat.

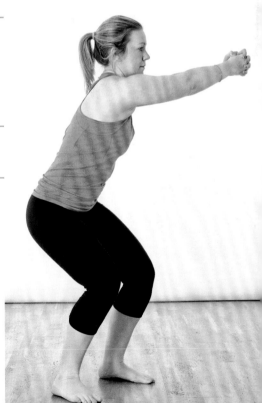

straight arm circle

17

Version 1

- Stand with your legs shoulder-width apart.

- Begin with your arms straight with your hands clasped together and in front of your hips.

- Draw the biggest imaginary circle you possibly can. Rotate right out to the side, as far above your head as you can then around to the other side.

- Finish with your arms back where they started and facing the floor again.

- Repeat, going in the opposite direction.

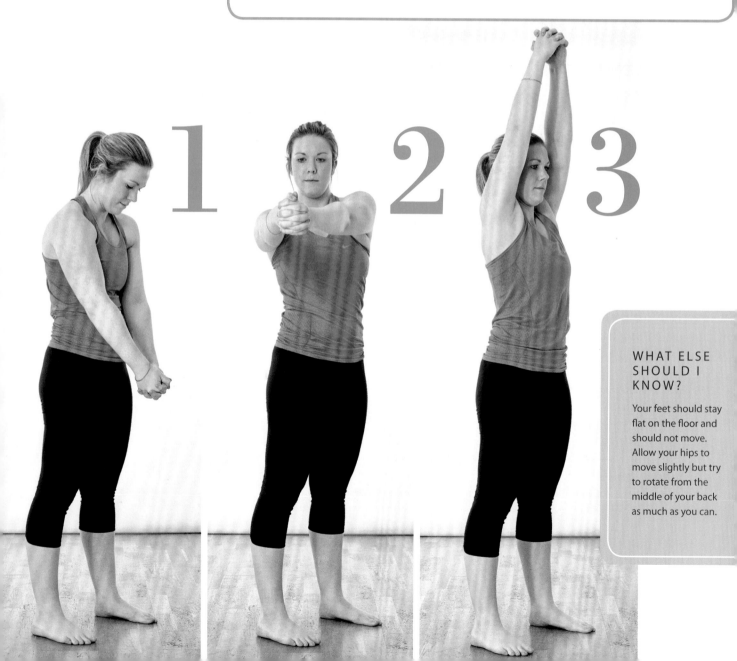

1   2   3

WHAT ELSE SHOULD I KNOW?

Your feet should stay flat on the floor and should not move. Allow your hips to move slightly but try to rotate from the middle of your back as much as you can.

Version 2

- Stand with your legs shoulder-width apart.

- Begin with your arms straight with your hands clasped together and in front of your hips.

- Bend your knees, going into a half squat so your hands are now closer to the floor.

- Extend your arms as far out to the side as you can as you push out from the half squat.

- Go right over your head and down the other side while moving back into the squat position.

- Finish with your arms back in position 1 and in the squat position.

- Repeat, going in the opposite direction.

WHAT ELSE SHOULD I KNOW?

This should be one long, fluid movement. Make sure you don't lean over as you extend your arms to the side. Remember to keep your feet flat on the floor and maintain a proper squat technique.

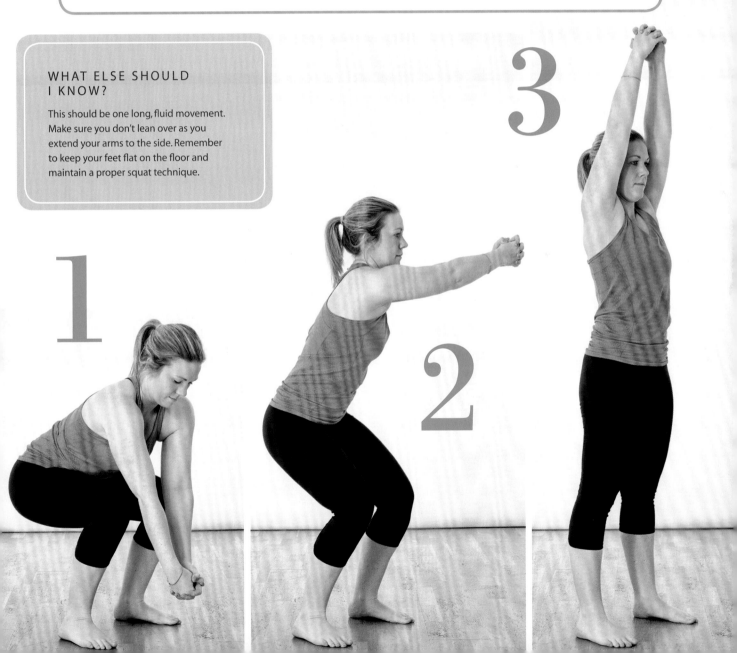

DAY 8

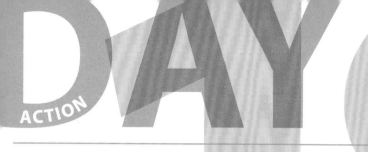

rest day

MUSCLES USED: None.

WHAT IT'S GOOD FOR? Chilling out, allowing your body to recover and grow.

WHY SHOULD YOU DO IT? Don't ignore muscles soreness as we're now beyond the halfway stage. Whether your body feels sore or not, why not head out for a walk today? Getting some fresh air in your lungs and some vitamin D-enriched sunlight for your skin will help to make you feel alive and ready to get back into it tomorrow.

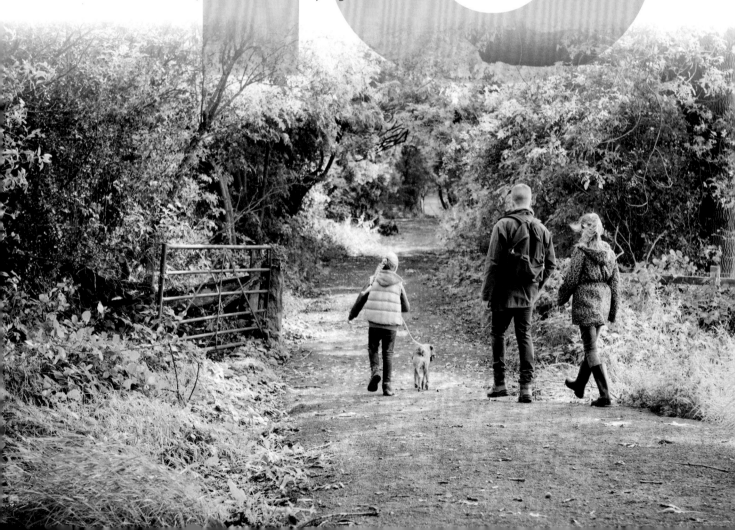

TODAY'S WORKOUT

PERFORM TODAY'S EXERCISE FOR 20 SECONDS, REST FOR 10 SECONDS AND REPEAT FOR 20 SECONDS. REST FOR 20 SECONDS BEFORE GOING BACK TO REPEAT YESTERDAY'S EXERCISE AND CONTINUE RIGHT BACK TO DAY 1.

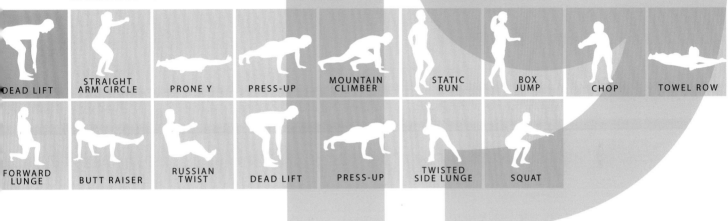

DEAD LIFT   STRAIGHT ARM CIRCLE   PRONE Y   PRESS-UP   MOUNTAIN CLIMBER   STATIC RUN   BOX JUMP   CHOP   TOWEL ROW

FORWARD LUNGE   BUTT RAISER   RUSSIAN TWIST   DEAD LIFT   PRESS-UP   TWISTED SIDE LUNGE   SQUAT

dead lift
(single leg dead lift)

REPEAT EXERCISE – SEE PAGE 119 FOR FULL DETAILS

WHY SHOULD YOU DO IT? You've been doing this exercise already since Day 4. This time, though, if you've been using both legs so far I'd like you to try and further challenge your core and balance by doing Version 2 (on one leg). This adds in a little rotation of your middle (something you're no doubt familiar with by now). When you're comfortable with the technique, why not try incorporating this exercise into your everyday life – each time you go to pick up something light from the floor, do it on one leg.

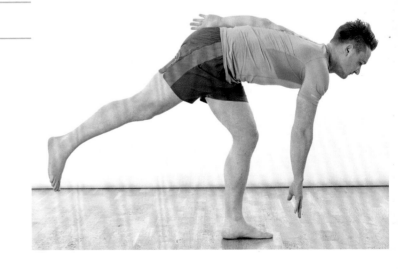

TODAY'S WORKOUT

PERFORM TODAY'S EXERCISE FOR 20 SECONDS, REST FOR 10 SECONDS AND REPEAT FOR 20 SECONDS. REST FOR 20 SECONDS BEFORE GOING BACK TO REPEAT YESTERDAY'S EXERCISE AND CONTINUE RIGHT BACK TO DAY 1.

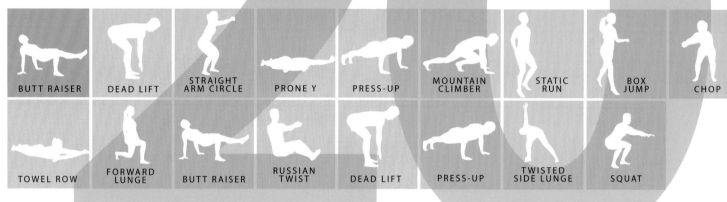

| BUTT RAISER | DEAD LIFT | STRAIGHT ARM CIRCLE | PRONE Y | PRESS-UP | MOUNTAIN CLIMBER | STATIC RUN | BOX JUMP | CHOP |

| TOWEL ROW | FORWARD LUNGE | BUTT RAISER | RUSSIAN TWIST | DEAD LIFT | PRESS-UP | TWISTED SIDE LUNGE | SQUAT |

butt raiser

REPEAT EXERCISE – SEE PAGE 128 FOR FULL DETAILS

WHY SHOULD YOU DO IT? 'Lazy butt syndrome' is one of the most common muscular problems I come across, so this is a really important exercise to include in your workout for a second time. By now though, your butt should be responding very well and this exercise ought to feel totally different the second time around. Putting it in again at this stage will also help you to properly engage your butt during all the exercises that follow. If up to now you've been sticking to Version 1, today could be the day you move on to Version 2. If, however you started out with Version 2 you can make this exercise more challenging by holding your position at the top for longer.

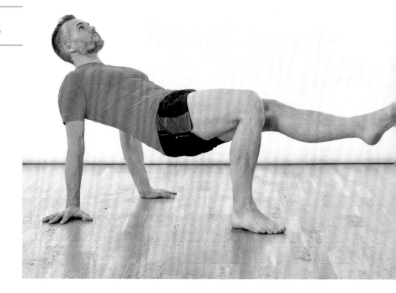

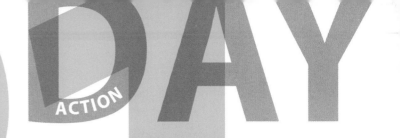

TODAY'S WORKOUT

PERFORM TODAY'S EXERCISE FOR 20 SECONDS, REST FOR 10 SECONDS AND REPEAT FOR 20 SECONDS. REST FOR 20 SECONDS BEFORE GOING BACK TO REPEAT YESTERDAY'S EXERCISE AND CONTINUE RIGHT BACK TO DAY 1.

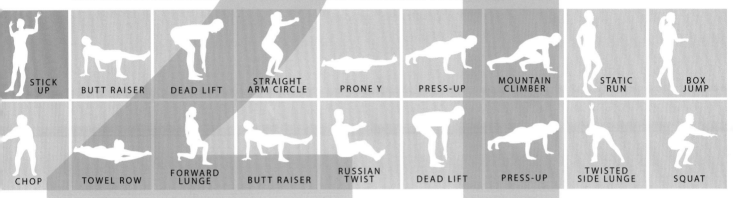

STICK UP | BUTT RAISER | DEAD LIFT | STRAIGHT ARM CIRCLE | PRONE Y | PRESS-UP | MOUNTAIN CLIMBER | STATIC RUN | BOX JUMP

CHOP | TOWEL ROW | FORWARD LUNGE | BUTT RAISER | RUSSIAN TWIST | DEAD LIFT | PRESS-UP | TWISTED SIDE LUNGE | SQUAT

stick-ups

MUSCLES USED: Trapezius/upper back, Deltoids/shoulders, Latissimus dorsi/middle back, Core.

WHAT IT'S GOOD FOR? Improving upper-body posture, throwing, flexibility, pulling, lifting, balancing things on your head (should you need to do so).

WHY SHOULD YOU DO IT? Remember those tricky Y shapes we made on Day 16? The stick-up builds on this and incorporates some core strength. This is all about improving your posture, which in turn saves other muscles from working more than they should (in particular your lower back). Try not to force this one though and don't be too surprised if you find it harder than you think it will be.

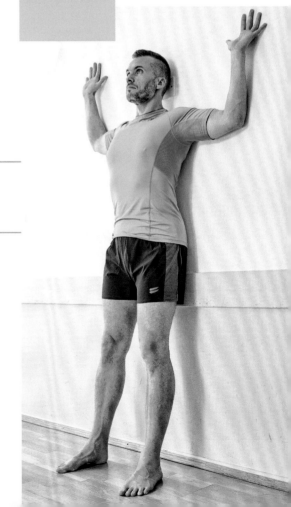

stick ups

Version 1

● Stand against a wall.

● Your butt and shoulders should be touching the wall throughout the whole exercise.

● Your heels should be about 10cm (4 inches) from the wall but your feet should remain flat on the floor throughout the whole exercise.

● Place the front of your arms on the wall and bend your elbows so your hands are in line with your shoulders and your fingers are pointing up. Your whole arm, shoulders and the back of your hands should be touching the wall.

● Slowly straighten your arms by pushing your hands up until they are above your head and touching each other. Your elbows and hands should still be in contact with the wall.

● Slowly return your arms back to the starting position.

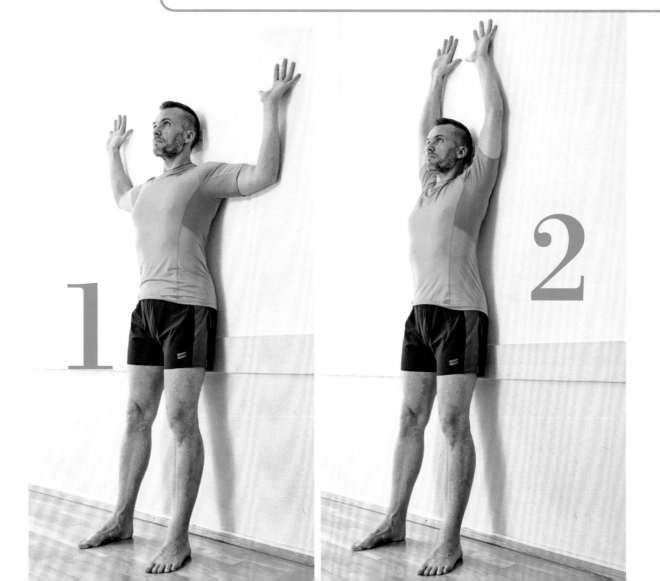

Version 2

- Stand against a wall.

- Your butt, shoulders and heels should be touching the wall throughout the whole exercise.

- Place the front of your arms on the wall and bend your elbows so your hands are in line with your shoulders and your fingers are pointing up. Your whole arm, shoulders and the back of your hands should be touching the wall.

- Slowly straighten your arms by pushing your hands up until they are above your head and touching each other. Your elbows and hands should still be in contact with the wall.

- Slowly return your arms back to the starting position.

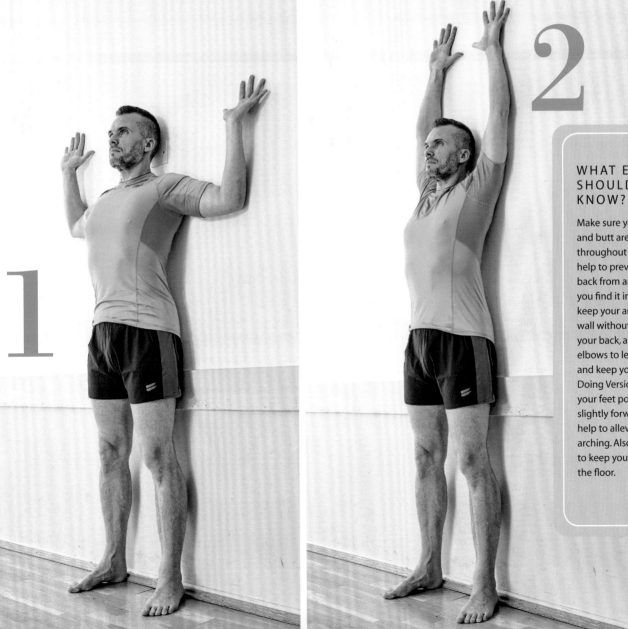

WHAT ELSE SHOULD I KNOW?

Make sure your core and butt are engaged throughout as this will help to prevent your back from arching. If you find it impossible to keep your arms on the wall without arching your back, allow your elbows to leave the wall and keep your back flat. Doing Version 1 with your feet positioned slightly forwards will help to alleviate the arching. Also remember to keep your feet flat on the floor.

TODAY'S WORKOUT

PERFORM TODAY'S EXERCISE FOR 20 SECONDS, REST FOR 10 SECONDS AND REPEAT FOR 20 SECONDS. REST FOR 20 SECONDS BEFORE GOING BACK TO REPEAT YESTERDAY'S EXERCISE AND CONTINUE RIGHT BACK TO DAY 1.

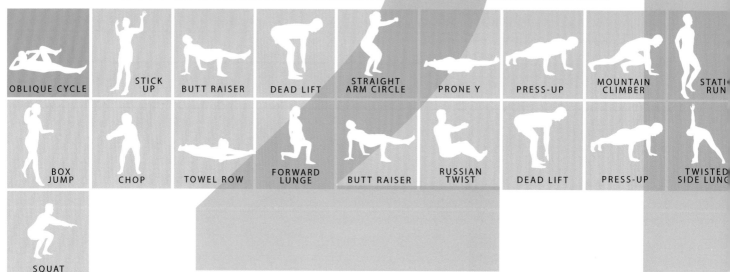

OBLIQUE CYCLE | STICK UP | BUTT RAISER | DEAD LIFT | STRAIGHT ARM CIRCLE | PRONE Y | PRESS-UP | MOUNTAIN CLIMBER | STATIC RUN

BOX JUMP | CHOP | TOWEL ROW | FORWARD LUNGE | BUTT RAISER | RUSSIAN TWIST | DEAD LIFT | PRESS-UP | TWISTED SIDE LUNGE

SQUAT

oblique cycle

MUSCLES USED: Obliques/side of core, Hip flexors, Latissimus dorsi/middle back.

WHAT IT'S GOOD FOR? Core strength, flexibility, coordination, running, racquet sports, any twisting movements.

WHY SHOULD YOU DO IT? This is a staple among traditional core exercises and, done properly, it can help to increase strength through the team of muscles that make up your core. By rotating through your middle you are placing emphasis on the muscles at your sides called obliques. These work to control this twisting movement, which we do countless times every day, such as when we unpack shopping from a car, load the dishwasher or do some gardening.

Version 1

- Lie on the floor with your elbows out to each side and your fingers touching your temples in front of your ears (not behind your head).

- Both legs should be off the floor with your right leg bent in and the left one straight.

- Lift your head off the floor and rotate your body anticlockwise until your right elbow reaches your right knee.

- Return to the starting position, and as you rotate in the opposite direction change legs so the left leg bends as the right one straightens.

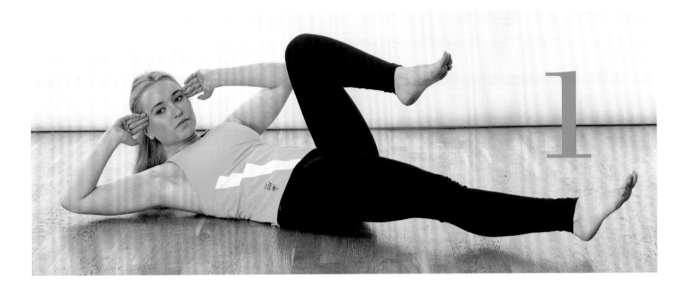

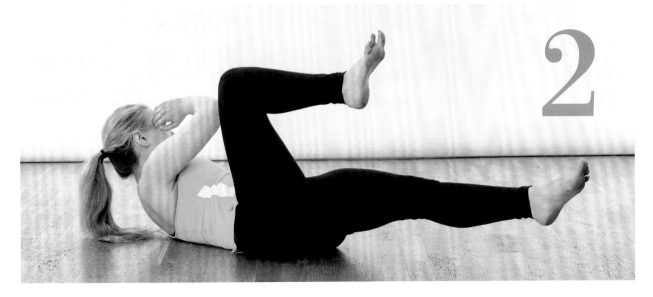

oblique cycle

Version 2

- Lie on the floor with your elbows out to each side and your fingers touching your temples in front of your ears (not behind your head).

- Both legs should be off the floor with your right leg bent in and the left one straight.

- Lift your head off the floor and rotate your body clockwise until your left elbow reaches your right knee.

- Return to the starting position, and as you rotate in the opposite direction change legs so the left leg bends as the right one straightens.

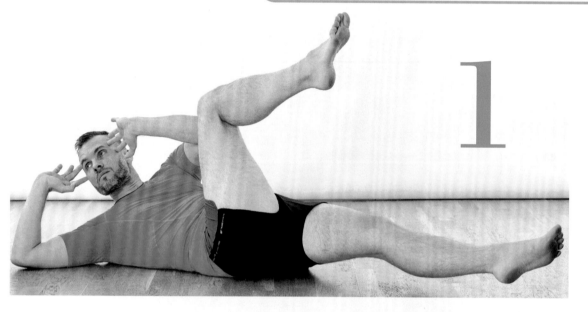

1

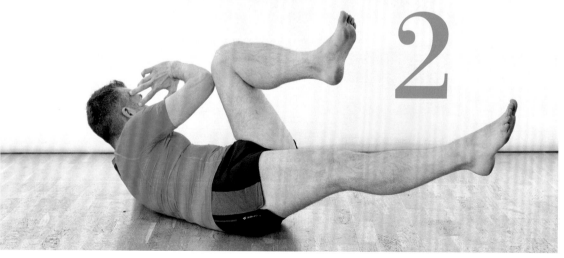

2

WHAT ELSE SHOULD I KNOW?

This whole exercise should be done at a speed you can control. It's very easy to pick up too much momentum. Version 1 slightly reduces the amount you need to rotate, which makes the exercise easier to manage as you get used to using your core for this movement. If you feel this in your lower back, your hips or the back of your neck, slow down or rest before having another go. It's quite common to suffer with pain in the back of your neck when performing exercises such as this. Remember, it works on core strength and flexibility, so try to focus your attention on your core and will the muscles around your middle to do the work for you.

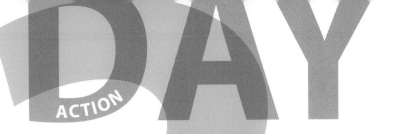

TODAY'S WORKOUT

PERFORM TODAY'S EXERCISE FOR 20 SECONDS, REST FOR 10 SECONDS AND REPEAT FOR 20 SECONDS. REST FOR 20 SECONDS BEFORE GOING BACK TO REPEAT YESTERDAY'S EXERCISE AND CONTINUE RIGHT BACK TO DAY 1.

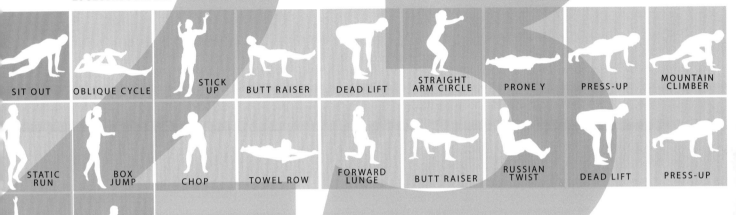

SIT OUT | OBLIQUE CYCLE | STICK UP | BUTT RAISER | DEAD LIFT | STRAIGHT ARM CIRCLE | PRONE Y | PRESS-UP | MOUNTAIN CLIMBER

STATIC RUN | BOX JUMP | CHOP | TOWEL ROW | FORWARD LUNGE | BUTT RAISER | RUSSIAN TWIST | DEAD LIFT | PRESS-UP

TWISTED SIDE LUNGE | SQUAT

sit out

MUSCLES USED: Quadriceps/thighs, Hamstrings, Gluteals/butt, Abductors/inside of thighs, Adductors/ outside of thighs, Obliques/side of core, Hip flexors, Latissimus dorsi/middle back, Core, Deltoids/shoulders, Triceps/back of arm.

WHAT IT'S GOOD FOR? Dance, racquet sports, golf, core strength, flexibility, coordination, running, any twisting movements.

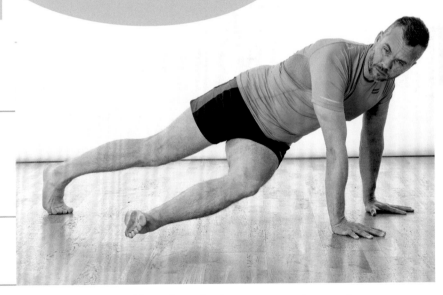

WHY SHOULD YOU DO IT? It's difficult to say what this exercise is *not* good for as it works almost every major muscle in your body and incorporates a very complex multi-directional movement pattern. It is particularly good for improving flexibility in your back, tests your balance and encourages your core to do the job it was really designed to do.

sit out

22

Version 1

- Start with your body facing the floor. Your arms should be straight and your hands on the floor directly underneath your shoulders. Your body needs to be straight with your feet behind you, hip-width apart, and your toes curled under.

- While maintaining this position, lift your left foot away from the floor, bend your left knee and twist your body so your left leg tucks underneath and extends straight out to your right.

- The outside of your left foot should end up on the floor, your hands should still be underneath your shoulders with your arms straight, and your butt should not be sticking up.

- Now bend your left leg again, draw it back under your body and return to the starting position.

- Repeat with the other leg.

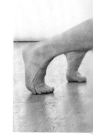

Version 2

- Start with your body facing the floor. Your arms should be straight and your hands on the floor directly underneath your shoulders. Your body needs to be straight with your feet behind you, hip-width apart, and your toes curled under.

- While maintaining this position, lift your left foot away from the floor, bend your left knee and twist your body so your left leg tucks underneath and extends straight out to your right.

- At the same time, take your right hand away from the floor. As you rotate towards the right your free arm should extend above you.

- Your supporting leg will now bend slightly as your hips lower towards the floor.

- Return straight back to the starting position and repeat in the opposite direction.

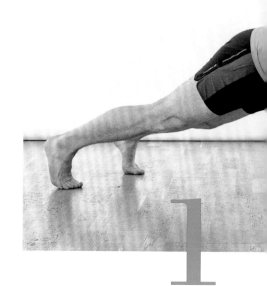

1

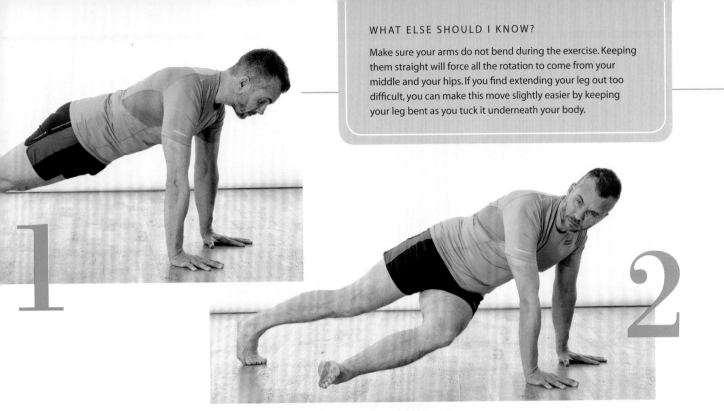

WHAT ELSE SHOULD I KNOW?

Make sure your arms do not bend during the exercise. Keeping them straight will force all the rotation to come from your middle and your hips. If you find extending your leg out too difficult, you can make this move slightly easier by keeping your leg bent as you tuck it underneath your body.

1

2

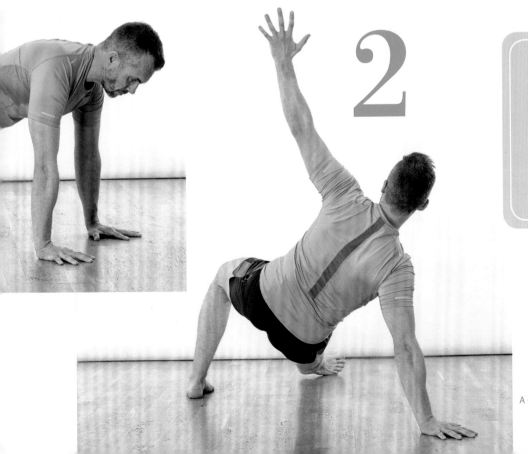

2

WHAT ELSE SHOULD I KNOW?

This harder version requires more stability and upper-body strength as you are supporting your upper bodyweight on just one arm. Make sure your supporting foot is flat on the floor at the end of the movement.

ACCUMULATOR ACTION **167**

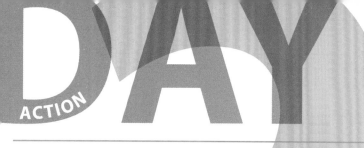

DAY 24

rest day

MUSCLES USED: None.

WHAT IT'S GOOD FOR? Relaxing, recovering and feeling generally good about yourself.

WHY SHOULD YOU DO IT? Just stop for a second and take a look at how far you've come. By now you will probably be doing things you have never done before and even though you may only have been regularly exercising for 24 days you will already be starting to feel a little different. It's important to listen to your body too though. If your muscles feel sore or tight, you will need to rest them (this may even take a couple of days, but that's fine). Exercising sore muscles can lead to injury so it's important to pay attention to them.

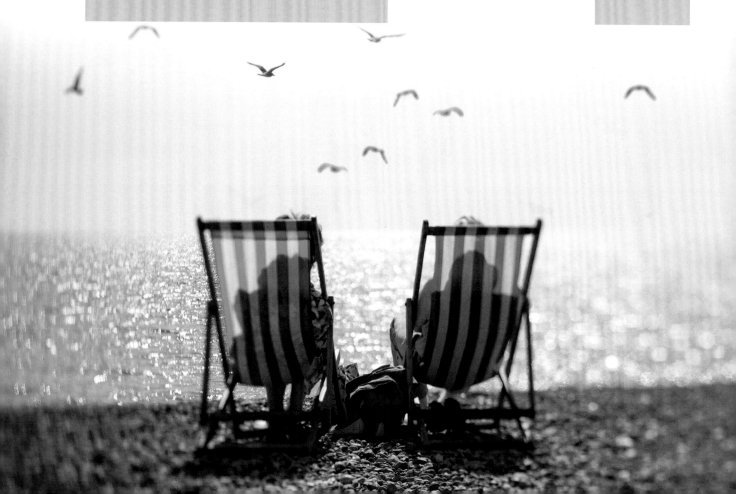

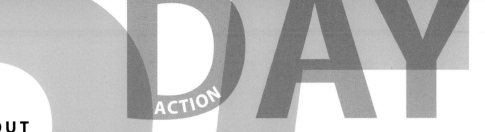

TODAY'S WORKOUT

PERFORM TODAY'S EXERCISE FOR 20 SECONDS, REST FOR 10 SECONDS AND REPEAT FOR 20 SECONDS. REST FOR 20 SECONDS BEFORE GOING BACK TO REPEAT YESTERDAY'S EXERCISE AND CONTINUE RIGHT BACK TO DAY 1.

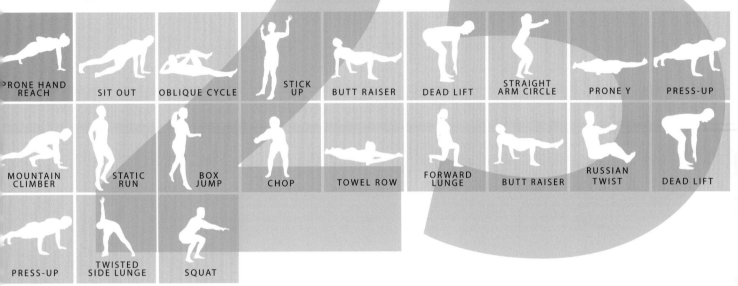

PRONE HAND REACH | SIT OUT | OBLIQUE CYCLE | STICK UP | BUTT RAISER | DEAD LIFT | STRAIGHT ARM CIRCLE | PRONE Y | PRESS-UP

MOUNTAIN CLIMBER | STATIC RUN | BOX JUMP | CHOP | TOWEL ROW | FORWARD LUNGE | BUTT RAISER | RUSSIAN TWIST | DEAD LIFT

PRESS-UP | TWISTED SIDE LUNGE | SQUAT

prone hand reach

MUSCLES USED: Gluteals/butt, Core, Deltoids/shoulders, Triceps/back of arm.

WHAT IT'S GOOD FOR? Core strength, stability.

WHY SHOULD YOU DO IT? This exercise is very good for properly activating all the muscles that make up your core. The more engaged your team of core muscles are, the more effective and safer all the other exercises in The Accumulator™ become (and a myriad of movements you make in everyday life). Many of us lack good core function because we sit down too much.

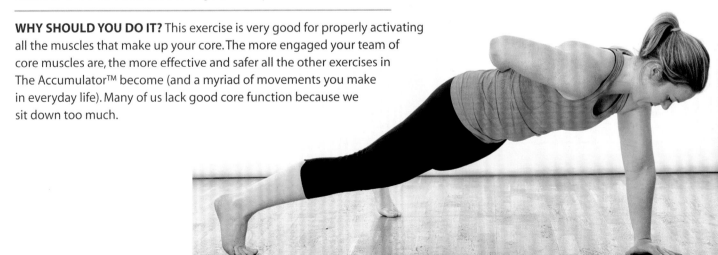

25

prone hand reach

Version 1

- Start with your body facing the floor. Your arms should be straight and your hands need to be on the floor in line with your shoulders but close enough together for your thumbs and index fingers to be touching each other.

- Your body should be straight with your feet behind you, and wider than your hips, with your toes curled under.

- Without moving any other part of your body, lift your left hand away from the floor and touch the top of your opposite shoulder.

- Return your hand to the floor and repeat with the other hand.

Version 2

- Start with your body facing the floor. Your arms should be straight and your hands need to be on the floor in line with your shoulders but close enough together for your thumbs and index fingers to be touching each other.

- Your body should be straight with your feet behind you, hip-width apart, with your toes curled under.

- Without moving any other part of your body, lift your left hand away from the floor and put it behind you so the front of your hand touches the middle of your back.

- Return your hand to the floor and repeat with the other hand.

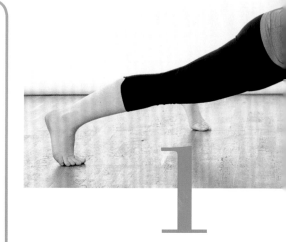

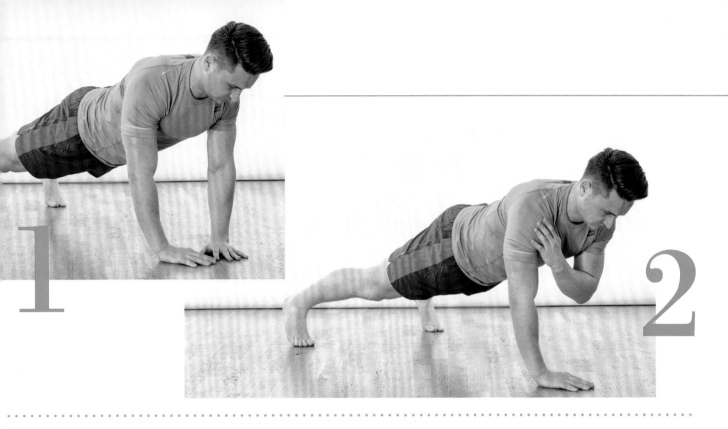

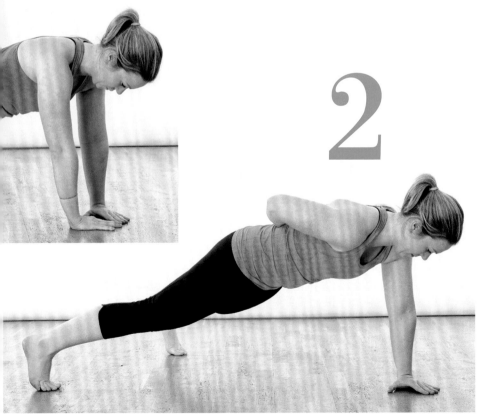

WHAT ELSE SHOULD I KNOW?

The objective here is to keep your hips perfectly still; they should not twist or lift. Imagine you have a tray of drinks on your back and try not to spill a drop. The further apart your feet are, the easier it will be to keep your hips still. The opposite applies to make the exercise harder. Think of your body like a tripod. The closer together the legs are the less stable you will become and therefore the harder your core has to work to stop you collapsing in a heap on the floor.

TODAY'S WORKOUT

PERFORM TODAY'S EXERCISE FOR 20 SECONDS, REST FOR 10 SECONDS AND REPEAT FOR 20 SECONDS. REST FOR 20 SECONDS BEFORE GOING BACK TO REPEAT YESTERDAY'S EXERCISE AND CONTINUE RIGHT BACK TO DAY 1.

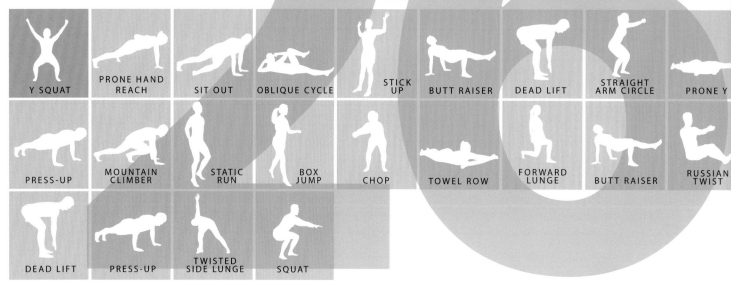

Y SQUAT	PRONE HAND REACH	SIT OUT	OBLIQUE CYCLE	STICK UP	BUTT RAISER	DEAD LIFT	STRAIGHT ARM CIRCLE	PRONE Y
PRESS-UP	MOUNTAIN CLIMBER	STATIC RUN	BOX JUMP	CHOP	TOWEL ROW	FORWARD LUNGE	BUTT RAISER	RUSSIAN TWIST
DEAD LIFT	PRESS-UP	TWISTED SIDE LUNGE	SQUAT					

Y squat

MUSCLES USED: Quadriceps/thighs, Gluteals/butt, Adductors/inside of thighs, Gastrocnemius/calves, Hamstrings, Illiopsoas/hip flexors, Core, Trapezius/upper back, Deltoids/shoulders, Latissimus dorsi/middle back.

WHAT IT'S GOOD FOR? Improving upper-body posture, throwing, flexibility, pulling, lifting, sitting down, jumping, running.

WHY SHOULD YOU DO IT? This is a combination of two exercises you have done before. The squat is a basic primal movement we do many times every day and there are numerous reasons why it's important for you to be able to do this with skill (see Day 1). Here, I've added in the Y shape we made on Day 16. This time, instead of facing the floor you stand so your own centre of gravity will challenge your upper-back strength as you go down for the squat.

Version 1

- Stand with your feet facing forwards, slightly wider than hip-width apart. Your big toes should be pointing roughly in the same direction as each other.

- Extend your arms above your head into a Y shape.

- Turn your hands around, make a fist and point your thumbs behind you. Keep your arms in exactly the same place for the whole exercise.

- Bend at the knees and hips as if you are about to sit in a chair.

- When your butt is at the same height as your knees, push yourself back up (by squeezing your butt).

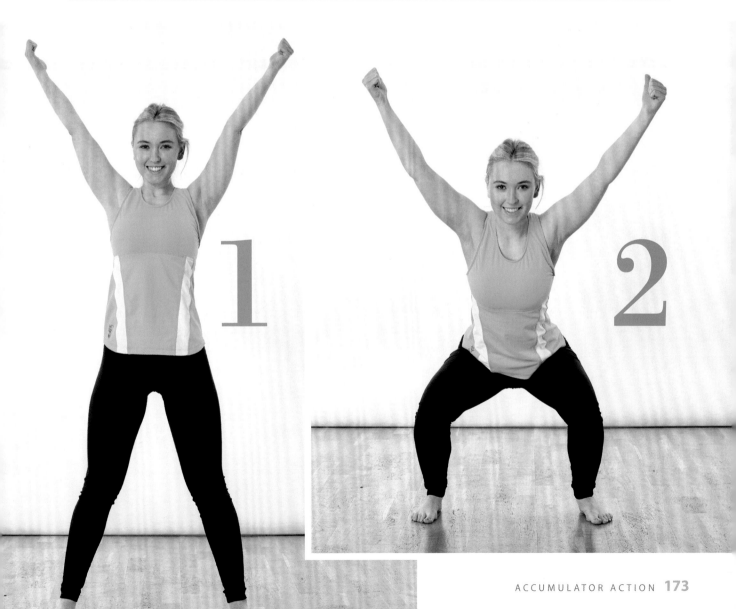

Y squat

Version 2

- Stand with your feet facing forwards, slightly wider than hip-width apart. Your big toes should be pointing in the same direction as each other.

- Extend your arms above your head into a Y shape.

- Turn your hands around, make a fist and point your thumbs behind you. Keep your arms in exactly the same place for the whole exercise.

- Bend at the knees and hips as if you are about to sit in a chair.

- Continue beyond knee height until the backs of your thighs touch your calves and your butt is close to the floor.

- Return to the starting position by squeezing your butt. Try to avoid the temptation to bounce back up.

WHAT ELSE SHOULD I KNOW?

Make sure your arms are above your head and not in front of it. Be careful not to arch your back as you squat. It's tempting to do this because your centre of gravity will change the lower you get. Because of this, the extra depth of the full squat in Version 2 will put more pressure on your arms and therefore make it harder to maintain the Y shape.

1

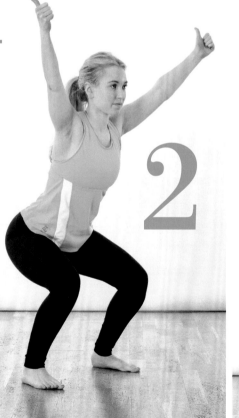

2

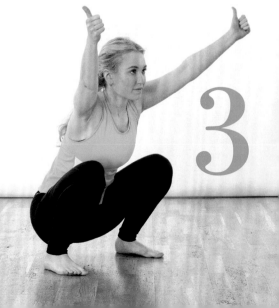

3

TODAY'S WORKOUT

PERFORM TODAY'S EXERCISE FOR 20 SECONDS, REST FOR 10 SECONDS AND REPEAT FOR 20 SECONDS. REST FOR 20 SECONDS BEFORE GOING BACK TO REPEAT YESTERDAY'S EXERCISE AND CONTINUE RIGHT BACK TO DAY 1.

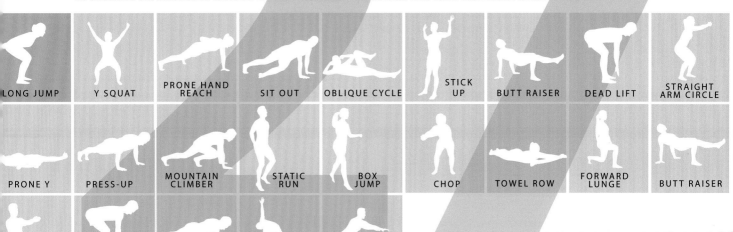

LONG JUMP | Y SQUAT | PRONE HAND REACH | SIT OUT | OBLIQUE CYCLE | STICK UP | BUTT RAISER | DEAD LIFT | STRAIGHT ARM CIRCLE

PRONE Y | PRESS-UP | MOUNTAIN CLIMBER | STATIC RUN | BOX JUMP | CHOP | TOWEL ROW | FORWARD LUNGE | BUTT RAISER

RUSSIAN TWIST | DEAD LIFT | PRESS-UP | TWISTED SIDE LUNGE | SQUAT

long jumps

MUSCLES USED: Quadriceps/thighs, Gluteals/butt, Adductors/inside of thighs, Gastrocnemius/calves, Hamstrings, Illiopsoas/hip flexors, Core.

WHAT IT'S GOOD FOR? Jumping, running, any sport requiring explosive movement, cardiovascular system.

WHY SHOULD YOU DO IT? This is known as a plyometric exercise, which indicates that it encourages your muscles to exert as much force as possible in short, explosive movements. This particular one is brilliant for improving power and flexibility in the muscles you use to run, in particular your calves and the muscles and tendons in your feet. If you have neighbours living underneath you, it might be an idea to let them know what you're up to before you start today.

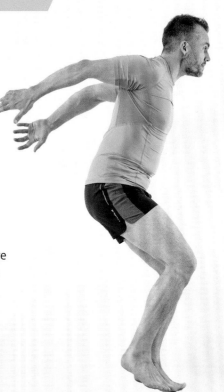

long jump

There is only 1 version today

● Stand with your feet facing forwards, slightly wider than hip-width apart. Your big toes should be pointing in the same direction as each other.

● Bend at the knees and hips as if you are about to sit in a chair. At the same time, send your arms behind you.

● As you push out of the squat, use your arms to propel you forwards and try to jump forwards as far as you can.

● At this point you have two options: if space is at a premium, you can simply step back and repeat the movement; if you have room, just keep going forwards.

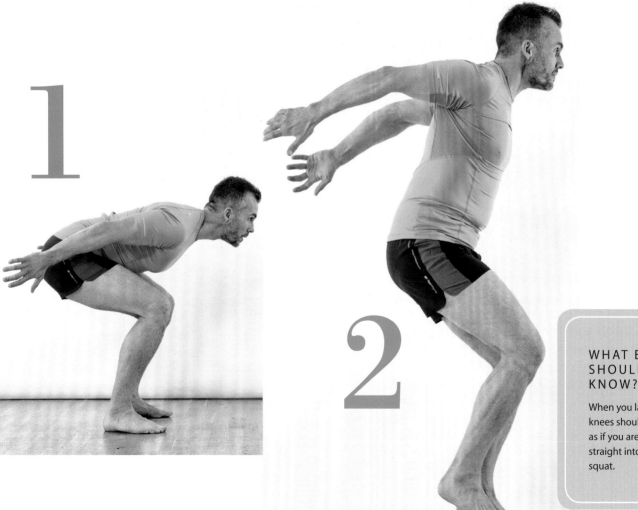

1

2

WHAT ELSE SHOULD I KNOW?

When you land your knees should be soft, as if you are heading straight into the next squat.

TODAY'S WORKOUT

PERFORM TODAY'S EXERCISE FOR 20 SECONDS, REST FOR 10 SECONDS AND REPEAT FOR 20 SECONDS. REST FOR 20 SECONDS BEFORE GOING BACK TO REPEAT YESTERDAY'S EXERCISE AND CONTINUE RIGHT BACK TO DAY 1.

PRESS-UP	LONG JUMP	Y SQUAT	PRONE HAND REACH	SIT OUT	OBLIQUE CYCLE	STICK UP	BUTT RAISER	DEAD LIFT
STRAIGHT ARM CIRCLE	PRONE Y	PRESS-UP	MOUNTAIN CLIMBER	STATIC RUN	BOX JUMP	CHOP	TOWEL ROW	FORWARD LUNGE
BUTT RAISER	RUSSIAN TWIST	DEAD LIFT	PRESS-UP	TWISTED SIDE LUNGE	SQUAT			

press-up (reverse press-up)

REPEAT EXERCISE – SEE PAGE 118 AND 148 FOR FULL DETAILS

WHY SHOULD YOU DO IT? We're going back to the same exercise we did on Day 15 today. There are a few good reasons why the press-up appears in the workout three times. First, it is perhaps the best upper-body exercise because it recruits many different muscles at once; second, you may already be seeing some improvement in your performance. Remember, there are actually three different versions of the press-up in this plan so if you started out doing the easiest version you may feel ready to try the next one. The press-up is a staple exercise. Some people learn to love them, some do not. However, nobody can deny how beneficial they are when they are performed correctly.

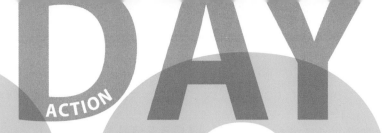

TODAY'S WORKOUT

PERFORM TODAY'S EXERCISE FOR 20 SECONDS, REST FOR 10 SECONDS AND REPEAT FOR 20 SECONDS. REST FOR 20 SECONDS BEFORE GOING BACK TO REPEAT YESTERDAY'S EXERCISE AND CONTINUE RIGHT BACK TO DAY 1.

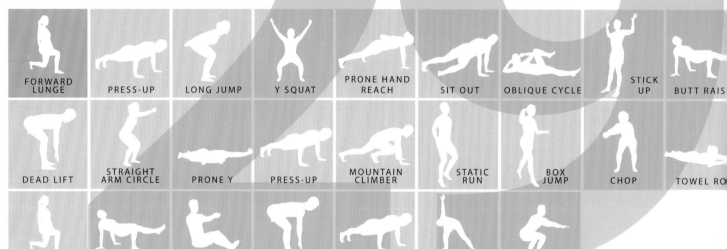

FORWARD LUNGE · PRESS-UP · LONG JUMP · Y SQUAT · PRONE HAND REACH · SIT OUT · OBLIQUE CYCLE · STICK UP · BUTT RAIS

DEAD LIFT · STRAIGHT ARM CIRCLE · PRONE Y · PRESS-UP · MOUNTAIN CLIMBER · STATIC RUN · BOX JUMP · CHOP · TOWEL RO

FORWARD LUNGE · BUTT RAISER · RUSSIAN TWIST · DEAD LIFT · PRESS-UP · TWISTED SIDE LUNGE · SQUAT

forward lunge
(prisoner lunge)

REPEAT EXERCISE – SEE PAGE 129 FOR FULL DETAILS

WHY SHOULD YOU DO IT? The lunge returns for a second appearance and, as with the press-up, at this stage of the month you may find the tight or inactive muscles that made the lunge hard at the start of the month will be limbering up and this exercise will be getting a little easier to do. If this is the case, try stepping things up a notch and having a go at Version 2.

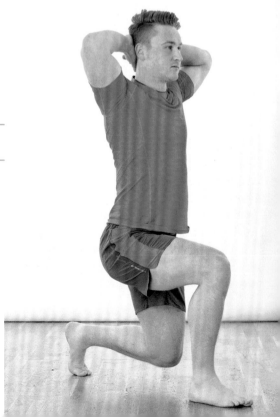

TODAY'S WORKOUT

PERFORM TODAY'S EXERCISE FOR 20 SECONDS, REST FOR 10 SECONDS AND REPEAT FOR 20 SECONDS. REST FOR 20 SECONDS BEFORE GOING BACK TO REPEAT YESTERDAY'S EXERCISE AND CONTINUE RIGHT BACK TO DAY 1.

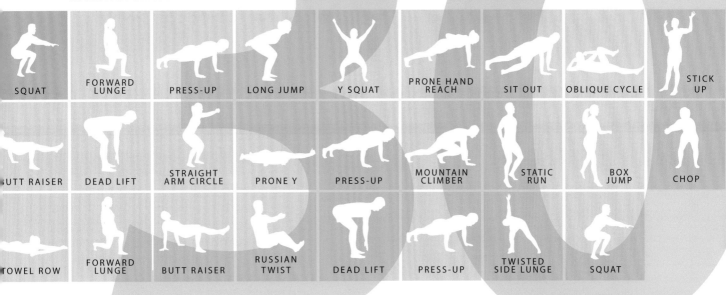

| SQUAT | FORWARD LUNGE | PRESS-UP | LONG JUMP | Y SQUAT | PRONE HAND REACH | SIT OUT | OBLIQUE CYCLE | STICK UP |

| BUTT RAISER | DEAD LIFT | STRAIGHT ARM CIRCLE | PRONE Y | PRESS-UP | MOUNTAIN CLIMBER | STATIC RUN | BOX JUMP | CHOP |

| TOWEL ROW | FORWARD LUNGE | BUTT RAISER | RUSSIAN TWIST | DEAD LIFT | PRESS-UP | TWISTED SIDE LUNGE | SQUAT |

squat

REPEAT EXERCISE – SEE PAGE 110 FOR FULL DETAILS

WHY SHOULD YOU DO IT? We finish right back where we started with the squat, one of the most important movements your legs and butt can do. With stretching and practice you may even find your squats are now closer to the floor than they were when you started.

WELL DONE! Now you've finished your first month using The Accumulator™. Don't stop there – have a look at pages 178–183 to find lots of ways you can make your workout more challenging again for another month. Alternatively, there are brand new workouts online at www.theaccumulator.net.

To make life easier, on the next page there's a list of the exercises which you can stick up on your wall.

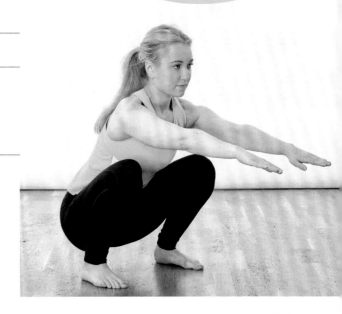

What can you do beyond 30 days?

SSO YOU'VE DONE ALL 30 DAYS OF THE ACCUMULATOR™ WORKOUT FEATURED IN THIS BOOK. NOW WHAT? THERE ARE A NUMBER OF WAYS YOU CAN CREATE A BRAND NEW WORKOUT USING ONLY THE EXERCISES FEATURED HERE. SIMPLY BY CHANGING THE ORDER OR INCREASING THE FREQUENCY THAT CERTAIN EXERCISES APPEAR CAN MAKE THE WORKOUT MUCH MORE OF A CHALLENGE AND WILL FURTHER TEST YOUR NEWLY IMPROVED FITNESS LEVELS.

In this chapter you can find 4 different ways to switch around the exercises in this book. You can also find many more workouts with brand new exercises on the website (www.theaccumulator.net).

Another simple way to increase the difficulty of the whole routine is by increasing the time you spend on each new exercise. So, instead of doing each exercise for 20 seconds twice with a 10 second interval, try one of these:

Exercise: 20 seconds.
Rest: 10 seconds.
Repeat the exercise: 20 seconds.
Rest: 10 seconds.
Repeat the exercise: 20 seconds.
Rest: 20 seconds.
Move on to next exercise.

Exercise: 30 seconds.
Rest: 20 seconds.
Repeat the exercise: 30 seconds.
Rest: 20 seconds.
Move on to next exercise.

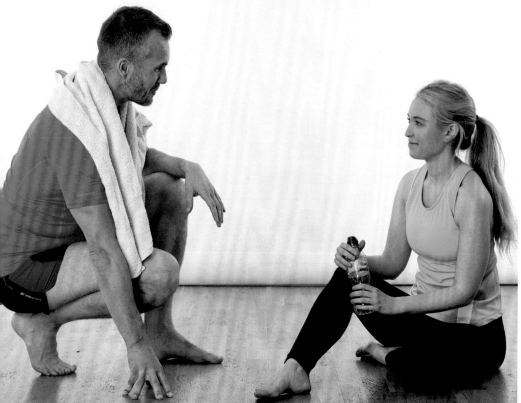

THE STANDARD ACCUMULATOR WORKOUT

DAY	EXERCISE	DAY	EXERCISE
1	SQUAT	16	PRONE Y
2	TWISTED SIDE LUNGE	17	STRAIGHT ARM CIRCLE
3	PRESS-UP	18	REST DAY
4	DEADLIFT	19	DEAD LIFT (SINGLE LEG DEAD LIFT)
5	RUSSIAN TWIST	20	BUTT RAISER
6	REST DAY	21	STICK-UPS
7	BUTT RAISER	22	OBLIQUE CYCLE
8	FORWARD LUNGE (PRISONER LUNGE)	23	SIT OUT
9	TOWEL ROLL	24	REST DAY
10	CHOP	25	PRONE HAND REACH
11	BOX JUMP	26	Y SQUAT
12	REST DAY	27	LONG JUMPS
13	STATIC RUN	28	PRESS-UP (REVERSE PRESS-UP)
14	MOUNTAIN CLIMBER	29	FORWARD LUNGE (PRISONER LUNGE)
15	PRESS-UP (REVERSE PRESS-UP)	30	SQUAT

THE REVERSE WORKOUT

DAY	EXERCISE	DAY	EXERCISE
1	SQUAT	16	PRESS-UP (REVERSE PRESS-UP)
2	FORWARD LUNGE (PRISONER LUNGE)	17	MOUNTAIN CLIMBER
3	PRESS-UP (REVERSE PRESS-UP)	18	STATIC RUN
4	LONG JUMPS	19	REST DAY
5	Y SQUAT	20	BOX JUMP
6	PRONE HAND REACH	21	CHOP
7	REST DAY	22	TOWEL ROW
8	SIT OUT	23	FORWARD LUNGE (PRISONER LUNGE)
9	OBLIQUE CYCLE	24	BUTT RAISER
10	STICK UPS	25	REST DAY
11	BUTT RAISER	26	RUSSIAN TWIST
12	DEAD LIFT (SINGLE LEG DEAD LIFT)	27	DEADLIFT
13	REST DAY	28	PRESS-UP (REVERSE PRESS-UP)
14	STRAIGHT ARM CIRCLE	29	TWISTED SIDE LUNGE
15	PRONE Y	30	SQUAT

THE ODDS AND EVENS

DAY	EXERCISE	DAY	EXERCISE
1	SQUAT	16	SQUAT
2	PRESS-UP (REVERSE PRESS-UP)	17	PRESS-UP
3	Y SQUAT	18	REST DAY
4	SIT OUT	19	RUSSIAN TWIST
5	STICK UP	20	FORWARD LUNGE (PRISONER LUNGE)
6	REST DAY	21	CHOP
7	DEAD LIFT (SINGLE LEG DEAD LIFT)	22	STATIC RUN
8	PRONE Y	23	PRESS-UP (REVERSE PRESS-UP)
9	MOUNTAIN CLIMBER	24	REST DAY
10	BOX JUMP	25	STRAIGHT ARM CIRCLE
11	TOWEL ROW	26	BUTT RAISER
12	REST DAY	27	OBLIQUE CYCLE
13	BUTT RAISER	28	PRONE HAND REACH
14	DEAD LIFT (SINGLE LEG DEAD LIFT)	29	LONG JUMP
15	TWISTED SIDE LUNGE	30	FORWARD LUNGE (PRISONER LUNGE)

UPPER AND LOWER

DAY	EXERCISE	DAY	EXERCISE
1	SQUAT	16	BOX JUMP
2	PRESS-UP (REVERSE PRESS-UP)	17	CHOP
3	LONG JUMPS	18	REST DAY
4	Y SQUAT	19	PRONE Y
5	BUTT RAISER	20	PRESS-UP (REVERSE PRESS-UP)
6	REST DAY	21	TOWEL ROW
7	PRESS-UP (REVERSE PRESS-UP)	22	RUSSIAN TWIST
8	PRONE HAND REACH	23	PRESS-UP (REVERSE PRESS-UP)
9	SIT OUT	24	REST DAY
10	OBLIQUE CYCLE	25	FORWARD LUNGE (PRISONER LUNGE)
11	STICK UPS	26	BUTT RAISER
12	REST DAY	27	DEAD LIFT (SINGLE LEG DEAD LIFT)
13	DEAD LIFT (SINGLE LEG DEAD LIFT)	28	TWISTED SIDE LUNGE
14	MOUNTAIN CLIMBER	29	SQUAT
15	STATIC RUN	30	CHOP

REPEATER (HARD)

DAY	EXERCISE	DAY	EXERCISE
1	SQUAT	16	TOWEL ROW
2	FORWARD LUNGE (PRISONER LUNGE)	17	TOWEL ROW
3	SQUAT	18	REST DAY
4	FORWARD LUNGE (PRISONER LUNGE)	19	PRONE HAND REACH
5	BUTT RAISER	20	OBLIQUE CYCLE
6	REST DAY	21	PRONE HAND REACH
7	BUTT RAISER	22	OBLIQUE CYCLE
8	DEAD LIFT (SINGLE LEG DEAD LIFT)	23	RUSSIAN TWIST
9	PRESS-UP (REVERSE PRESS-UP)	24	REST DAY
10	MOUNTAIN CLIMBER	25	LONG JUMP
11	PRESS-UP (REVERSE PRESS-UP)	26	BOX JUMP
12	REST DAY	27	MOUNTAIN CLIMBER
13	MOUNTAIN CLIMBER	28	STATIC RUN
14	Y SQUAT	29	TWISTED SIDE LUNGE
15	Y SQUAT	30	TWISTED SIDE LUNGE

Don't take my word for it ...

GILLIAN ANDERSON

Before discovering The Accumulator™ I was a regular in the gym, sticking mainly to the treadmill, the cross trainer and a few weights – all the usual stuff. But I found I was getting stuck in a rut and I was just doing the same old thing all the time, which was becoming boring. I'm retired and in the fortunate position of being able to have lots of holidays, but I always found it hard to get enough exercise in when I was away. Then, on New Year's Day, I was visiting a friend of my sister-in-law and she mentioned she was taking part in The Accumulator™. So I decided to give it a go too.

Straight away I found I really enjoyed the variety of exercises and the way the workout plan grows throughout the month. The big advantage for me though is that The Accumulator™ is completely mobile, so I always have it.

Sometimes when I'm away in a hotel the gym may not be great (if there is one), so it's nice to know that I've always got a plan and I can do the routine every day, regardless of where I am.

As each month progresses I'm always amazed by the improvement I'll make doing the exercises that appeared early on in the month. As I've been taking part for a year now, sometimes exercises I've done in previous months will re-appear and although the first time around they may have been hard, now they are easier; I can really see how much my strength and stamina have improved. As I had been going to the gym for so long before doing The Accumulator™ I didn't think it would make a massive difference to me, but it really has. My core strength is much better than it has ever been and my running is much faster too. I had a shoulder injury many years ago so my left arm had always been weak, but I can really see and feel a difference there too – I can do a lot more with it now.

Earlier this year I took part in a trek through the Andes and along the Inca trail. There was a lot of steep climbing to do, which is not only tough on the legs and bum but also

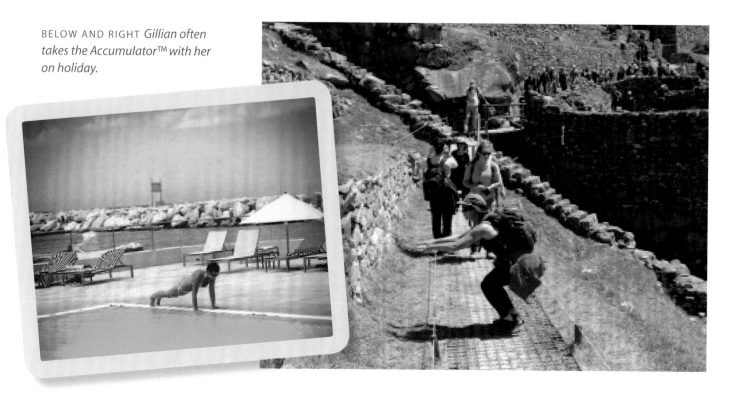

BELOW AND RIGHT *Gillian often takes the Accumulator™ with her on holiday.*

requires a lot of strength in the back and shoulders because you use poles to pull yourself up. The other people on our trip were all experienced trekkers and at first they were horrified to have novices in their group, until they started struggling to keep up because being fitter and stronger was much more important than being experienced. They would spend every evening and morning complaining about how sore their legs and backs were, but mine were fine. The advantages I had on this trip I owe entirely to The Accumulator™.

I think The Accumulator™ works on lots of different levels for many different people. For me, it started out as a supplement and now it helps me to do all the things I enjoy, such as running and walking. I actually do very few weights in the gym these days, because I don't feel I need to. The definition and strength I have built up is as a result of the bodyweight exercises I have done with The Accumulator™ and not thanks to dumb-bells or bar-bells. Before I started I would not have thought it was possible to change my body as much as I have using only my bodyweight. It's weird, because after doing the first month I did wonder what the point of doing it continuously would be as you go back to a single exercise on Day 1 when you start afresh. But it works, and I like that part now because the final week of the month is really intense as the workouts get longer. Starting again gives my body the chance to recover and, because it begins gradually I can see how great The Accumulator™ is for people who are starting out and are not as fit as me. I think many of my friends assume it's really hard because I've always loved exercise and therefore wouldn't do something that was easy.

MELANIE SMITH

Before doing The Accumulator™ I couldn't stick at anything. I did a little swimming but couldn't keep it up because of childcare issues or work commitments. Then I tried running for a few weeks and hated it – I felt so puffed out and paranoid running around in the unprofessional-looking gear I was wearing. So I got bored and stopped. It's a good job my work as a gardener is very active otherwise I would've been overweight, but since I had done physical work for years I think my body had stopped classing it as exercise and it wasn't enough to keep me really fit.

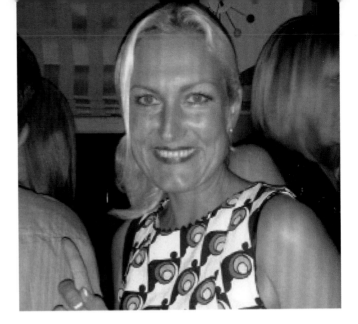

ABOVE *Melanie Smith. "The Accumulator™ has changed my body all over".*

I never really thought I would find something that worked, but then one day my old school friend, Leah, asked if I wanted to try The Accumulator™. I remember Day 1 was a plank. I was rather wobbly then and hated looking down at my stomach flesh hanging in a triangle. That plank was hard too. I think The Accumulator™ was the kick up the backside this girl needed. So I got a grip of myself.

The Accumulator™ has changed my body all over – arms, legs, bum, and my abs have real tone too. I can see the makings of a six-pack and if I ate properly instead of scoffing doughnuts and pastries I think I could actually have one. I also find my moods are much better when I exercise and I naturally eat better – because it gives me a focus for the day, I'm less tempted to plunge my hand into the cookie jar.

I do The Accumulator™ at various times, depending on how the day goes. But that's the great thing: you can squeeze it in whenever you like. Some days I have done it at 11.30 p.m. and others first thing in the morning. But I always find time to get it done. I have done fitness DVDs in the past too, but found that if I am the instigator of the exercise or have to press 'play' on my own it's almost like my motivation evaporates. I am extremely happy to have found The Accumulator™ and such a fantastic group of people. It's a great connection.

MOIRA TAYLOR

I have always been into my exercise and before taking on The Accumulator™ I was already doing two or three classes each week with Paul as well as walking the dog (without Paul). The classes were really working and I felt so much fitter and more toned from working with Paul.

When Paul first told me about The Accumulator™, my previous experience of him as such a great teacher made me sign up straight away. It's a really challenging way to exercise and I often get the whole family involved. This makes it much more fun than going out to the dreaded gym, as well as being so much better than any workout you would ever do by yourself. Once I start, I'm hooked in and my mental strength, along with the lack of time to hang about, sees me to the end every time.

I really like the structure and it's relatively quick – not simple, but quick. This way of working out suits me perfectly and I can easily fit it in around my busy family and work life. The Accumulator™ is much more me than any workout DVD as all the glamour has been taken out (sorry Paul). Unlike so many of those fitness DVDs, this is more about the exercises and how they benefit you than how you look. There's also no dancing or side-stepping in sight.

JULIA IBBITSON

I used to be very active years ago but more recently had lost motivation and I found that I needed something new to inspire me. A few years ago I regularly did classes, swam and ran. I worked 9–5 then, so it was much easier, but once I qualified as a nurse I began to struggle to find a routine that would fit around shifts and working long hours. I used to love the gym and would probably describe myself as having been addicted, so when I couldn't make time to maintain the level of fitness I had previously enjoyed I became a little despondent.

The Accumulator™ changed all that, and it is easy to fit around my shifts although sometimes towards the end of the month I have to shuffle a little as I don't always feel like doing much after a busy 12–14-hour shift. I have a spare room I use to exercise in, although my family have got used to me jumping around the living room on occasion.

I have felt fitter since taking part too. I have lost a stone without too many changes to my diet and have definitely

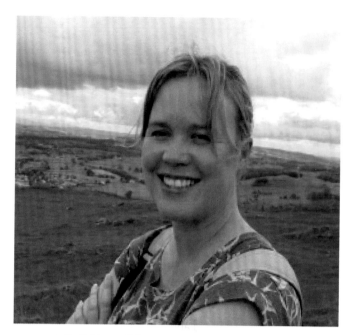

ABOVE *Julia Ibbitson. "I lost a stone without too many changes to my diet".*

noticed that my arms are becoming more toned. I also feel less tired when working busy shifts and the workout plan has boosted my self-confidence too. I have bought DVDs in the past, done them a couple of times and then left them gathering dust. The beauty of The Accumulator™ is that you are not doing it on your own, so you are more likely to stick to it.

SIMON THOMAS

Before The Accumulator™ I wasn't really doing that much. Unfortunately, my rugby days are behind me, but during my regular gym visits in the past I used to focus on aerobic or semi-aerobic exercises. I have always struggled to motivate myself to do resistance training, and used my larger frame as an excuse not to do bodyweight activities. In recent years, work has become busier and kids have arrived, making demands on my time, so I have done less and less. I had to give up my gym membership because I couldn't find the time to go, and so I bought home equipment, which quickly became a bit boring. I tried running, but a year ago developed Achilles tendonitis so I had to drop that. I enjoy exercising, which made my inability to find the time doubly upsetting. I saw myself gaining weight and losing fitness (I used to be the fittest on the rugby pitch, but I started feeling my body reverberate if I went for a gentle jog).

So, I took the plunge, started The Accumulator™ and discovered that I love it. Going to the gym, or even doing a home exercise session can often mean an hour's work with more time getting changed and showering afterwards. As a result, if I couldn't afford to devote two hours to working out in the evening, I would do nothing. With The Accumulator™ I do something every day, even if not for very long. The fact that it is more resistance-based means that even 5–10 minutes can lead to a sweat.

The biggest benefit for me though is that it's so easy mentally to start an exercise session ('10 minutes is all I need, of course I can do tonight'). Then, once I've got going, adding to it becomes easier ('well, I'm changed now and have got up a bit of a sweat – I might as well do another 10 minutes on the rower').

When the workout is quick (e.g. for the first week) I will often do it before I go to work, but after then I usually try to do it in the evening. That way it can also lead to a longer session if I feel motivated enough. My children sometimes do it with me too and it's quite nice to have them do some exercise alongside – it gives me a chance to give them some advice.

It's a very useful exercise workout in that it doesn't require any equipment. I have been able to do it in hotel rooms when I have been away on work trips, or even holidays. I am fortunate enough to live in Stirling, Scotland, which means that we quite often go hill walking, and within a couple of hours from home we are on the top of a Munro (the name for a mountain in Scotland). The views from up there are definitely conducive to a few squats or press-ups.

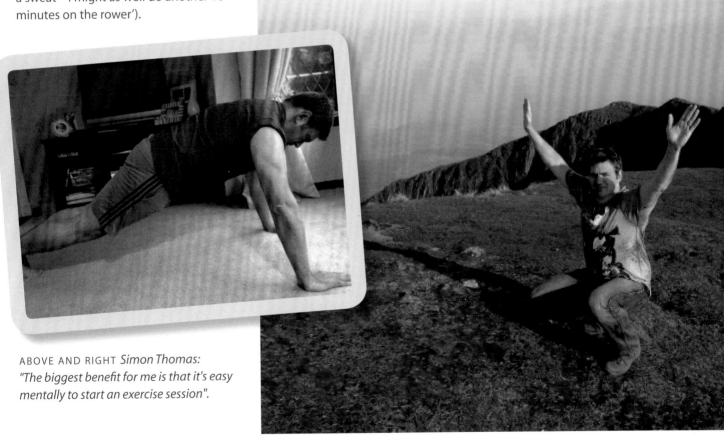

ABOVE AND RIGHT *Simon Thomas:*
"The biggest benefit for me is that it's easy mentally to start an exercise session".

Index

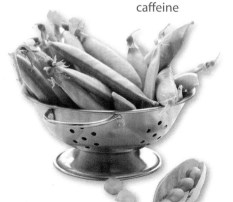

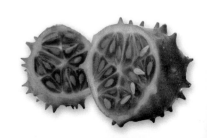

Acknowledgements

I'll readily admit I never read this part of a book because it usually contains a long list of people I don't know but please read it. I'm not going to run down a long list of people here but I do really need to thank some people for their help in the making of this book and I hope you will indulge me by taking a look.

Professionally there are a number of people over the years who have inspired me, taught me and without whom I would not have known any of this information I am passing on to you. So actually you owe them some thanks too. Among those who really deserve a mention here are Mike Nicholls, Mark Pryke, Nichola Curran, Ken Bob Saxton, Matthew Wallden and Linda Perkins. I should also thank every single person I have ever coached during the 10 years I have been working in the industry as they have all taught me to become a better coach. For their help with this book, thanks go to my models Laura Noble, Jack Mahoney and James St Pierre. I also owe a large thank you (and probably a hearty meal) to John Shepherd as without him I wouldn't have written this book in the first place. Finally and most importantly, a massive thank you to Emily Thompson who has been a huge help with The Accumulator™ since day one.

Personally I owe heaps to my wife Bridget and daughter Kyra for their patience while I locked myself in my office typing all these words and for the many hours I have spent working to develop The Accumulator™ concept.

Most importantly I have to thank and would like to dedicate this book to my Father, Maurice Mumford who sadly lost his battle with Motor Neurone Disease during the writing of this book. It was his love of fitness that started this whole journey to begin with and his financial input that made The Accumulator™ what it is today.

Our models are wearing clothes by Tribesports and Ilu Fitwear.

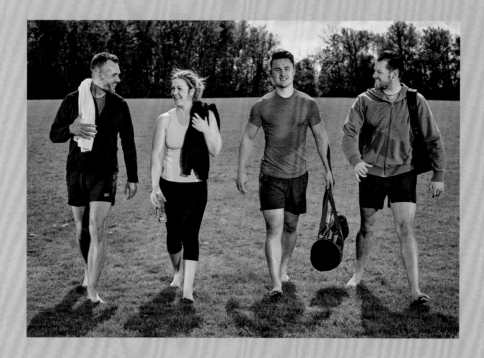